Living It Out

A survival guide for lesbian, gay and bisexual Christians and their friends, families and churches

Rachel Hagger-Holt
and Sarah Hagger-Holt

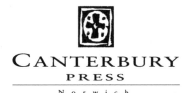

CANTERBURY
PRESS

Norwich

© Rachel Hagger-Holt and Sarah Hagger-Holt 2009

First published in 2009 by the Canterbury Press Norwich
Editorial office
13–17 Long Lane,
London, EC1A 9PN, UK

Canterbury Press is an imprint of Hymns Ancient and Modern Ltd
(a registered charity)
St Mary's Works, St Mary's Plain,
Norwich, NR3 3BH, UK

www.scm-canterburypress.co.uk

British Library Cataloguing in Publication data

A catalogue record for this book is available
from the British Library

978 1 85311 999 6

Typeset by Regent Typesetting, London
Printed and bound in Great Britain by
CPI William Clowes, Beccles NR34 7TL

Contents

Acknowledgements

In addition to our 54 contributors, there are many other fantastic people who have made it possible for us to complete *Living It Out*.

We'd like to thank these groups for letting us use their networks to advertise for contributors: Changing Attitude, Courage, Friends and Families of Lesbians and Gays (FFLAG), Inclusive Church, Women and the Church (WATCH) and Young LGBT Christians (YLGC).

Kind friends agreed to read through draft chapters, offering helpful comments and bringing new insights. These include: Bill, Catherine Barber, Elaine Ewart, Leigh-Anne Stevenson, Louise Palmer, Mark Burr, Richard Powell, Rob Harrison, Sarah Cantwell and Terry Biddington. We also greatly benefited from the help of Daniel Hale and Sophie Manuel, who bravely read through the entire book and offered feedback. Helen Bilton expertly compiled the index.

We'd like to pay tribute to Jon Birch, the man behind http://asbojesus.wordpress.com, whose thoughtful and funny cartoons you'll find scattered throughout this book. And to thank Chris Dicken for his technical and creative skills in helping us set up www.livingitout.com. Thanks to Alex Huzzey and David Warren for their encouragement and for allowing us to put finishing touches to several chapters from the comfort of their kitchen and using their laptops. Thanks also are due to Christine Smith and Canterbury Press for believing in *Living It Out*, helping shape and improve it and enabling it to reach a much wider audience.

Most of all, we owe a huge debt of gratitude to Vivien and Chris Holt who looked after us, fed and watered us, and entertained our daughter weekend after weekend as we sat and wrote in their conservatory. We promise we'll still come and visit even now we've finished the book.

We have used the New International Version when quoting verses from the Bible.

Introduction

Sarah

This is the book I wanted to read when I was 19.

It was the late 1990s. I'd come home after hearing a talk put on by my university Christian Union called 'Was Jesus anti-gay?' The room had been full and brightly lit. I'd sat at the back at the end of a row, ready to bolt for the door, and wondered if everyone else there cared as much about the answer to this question as I did. The speaker was a man who had 'overcome his homosexuality' and was now happily married to a woman and had two children. The message I'd taken home was that while Jesus may not be anti-gay, the rest of the church certainly could be.

I was now faced with a choice. I already knew how important my faith was to me and how I couldn't imagine life without it and I had now heard from someone who had made the decision to deny his sexual orientation, even leaving a relationship with another man, in order to follow God. Yet I knew deep down that this wasn't the right choice for me.

As far as I was aware, I didn't know any other lesbian, gay and bisexual (LGB) people, let alone any LGB Christians, but I knew that I wanted to. I wanted to see if there was a way of reconciling both parts of myself, to live well as a gay Christian, and if there was, I wanted to grab it with both hands.

Rachel

This is the book I never thought we'd actually write.

It's now 2007. Sarah and I are just home from work, and are eating dinner together. I mention casually, 'I was thinking, we should write a book.' This is the latest of many thoughts I've had, and Sarah usually provides the voice of reason. Just a few weeks before, I had idly wondered if God was calling us to move to New Zealand, as everywhere we looked there seemed to be posters, adverts and media articles all about the country. Sarah pointed out that there was much more about Iraq in the news than New Zealand, and if I wasn't willing to consider moving there, then maybe it wasn't God at all. But this time, her face brightens: 'Good idea! Let's start planning.'

And so, a day later, we have a huge Gantt chart made from sheets of A4 paper plastered across one wall of our study, and we're emailing everyone we know to see if they want to be involved . . .

Sarah and Rachel
Living It Out bears witness to the many LGB people we have met during the last ten years who hold an active faith, lived out in their daily lives.

Alongside them and thanks to them, we have renewed relationships with God and with the Bible, negotiated our paths through church, and continue to learn and grow in our Christian faith through good times and bad. They have helped us strive to live life well as Christians who are gay.

How can we all benefit from their experiences and their wisdom? We've found Bible commentaries from different perspectives, books of triumph or of pain from LGB people struggling with their sexual orientation and strident statements from pro- and anti-LGB Christian activists. But very little has been written about how to negotiate this sometimes contradictory yet enriching combination of identities. Where are the books sharing our stories, and those of our families, friends and churches?

Stories from people like Christine or Bruce, Christian parents whose understanding of the world was turned upside down when their children came out as gay. Or from straight Christians like Sophie whose faith found a new direction through sharing experiences with her LGB friends. Or from

LGB people like Kate who came out before finding faith. From ministers like Terry, wondering how to best support LGB people in their congregations. Or those like Anthony, considering how to answer a call to the ministry. We also wanted to hear the voices of people like 16-year-old Reuben, discovering how his teachers and classmates react to his sexual orientation or, like Paul T, who can look back on decades of partnership.

These are all people who have helped us to write this book. It includes their experiences, advice and stories and those of around 50 others (find out about them all on pages xii–xvi). They span at least eight denominations, and range in age from under 18 to over 70. We are incredibly grateful to every one of them for their honesty and their willingness to share sometimes very personal thoughts and feelings.

You can read *Living It Out* from cover to cover, or you can dip in wherever it most interests you. Each chapter deals with a different theme but follows a similar pattern, always ending with a suggested action and short prayer. All include quotes and stories from a variety of people, many of whom will become familiar as their stories thread through several different chapters. There are a few special features as well, which allow for more in-depth reflection from one person on an area not covered in the other chapters.

We felt it important to begin by thinking about ways of relating to God, so Chapter 1 explores how different people have responded to the deep-seated desire to know and be known by God. Next we face the Bible, often interpreted in ways that have prevented LGB people and their allies from relating to God and to other Christians. There can be a great deal of pain bound up in our relationship with 'the good book'. Yet despite the difficulties that many encounter, the Bible remains a source of inspiration and encouragement.

Our relationships with God and with the Bible are not worked out in isolation but in community, by sharing insights, praying and living alongside each other. So this is where the focus of the next four chapters lies: beginning with the difficulty of deciding 'Should I stay or should I go?' in a particular church and the struggles and joys of 'Coming out in church'; moving on to a discussion of family relationships and 'Family values' and finally exploring the role that joining groups plays in helping people to feel that they are 'No longer the only one'.

Chapters 7 and 8 cover 'Career path Christianity' and 'Love and marriage'. The issues of same-sex relationships and of the ministry of LGB people touch the very heart of people's lives and identities, and perhaps for that reason they have been deeply problematic for the institutional church. And finally, 'Speaking out' suggests positive, practical ways that we can continue to live out our faith as LGB Christians, families, friends and churches.

There is so much miscommunication and mistrust between people who hold different views about LGB issues both inside and outside the church. Rumour, stereotype and media sensationalism shape what we expect people who hold different views to us to be like. By sharing real people's stories, in all their complexity, we've tried to avoid the stereotypes of bigoted homophobes waving 'God hates fags' placards, and of promiscuous drag queens draped in rainbow flags, and instead to provide a place where 'LGB' and 'Christian' can sit happily side by side.

We hope that *Living It Out* speaks to you, however different your story may be from any of the ones here. You won't find definite answers or people telling you exactly how to live your life, but we hope that the insights and experiences of those who have walked a similar path will be of value. You'll also read some of our own stories and find out more about our church backgrounds during the course of *Living It Out*. We have tried to avoid our own experiences and assumptions colouring the book, but accept that this is inevitable. So for the times where we might have misunderstood or misrepresented traditions or viewpoints which are not our own, we apologize.

We've used 'you' throughout the text and have tried to be as inclusive as possible when doing so. But there will be lots of different readers who pick up this book, and this might mean that sometimes you feel that we are making assumptions about you or that we are talking to someone completely different. If so, please bear with us. And while we're on the subject of language, you might notice that we have tried to use LGB (standing for Lesbian, Gay and Bisexual) throughout. Although it can be clumsy, it is currently the clearest and most widely accepted term around. Similarly, despite its limitations, we have used the word 'straight' to refer to people who do not define themselves as LGB. The only exceptions are when quoting other people, where we have kept the language that they have used.

Although the internet has made it much easier for LGB Christians, their friends and their families, to meet each other, many still feel as isolated and alone as Sarah did at 19. One of the reasons behind *Living It Out* is to show people that they are not alone, that there are others living it out and that by sharing, laughing and crying together we can grow and flourish as loved children of God.

If you want to add your comments, find out more about this book or access further sources of support and information, we'd love to meet you at www.livingitout.com.

List of contributors

You will hear the voices of many different people speaking through the pages of *Living It Out*. Their stories, experiences and advice have made this book possible. To acknowledge their huge contribution – and because we thought you might want to know a little more about them – they are all introduced below. They describe themselves in their own words and are listed alphabetically by first name. We are very grateful to each of them and recognize that some have taken a personal risk in having their words quoted.

There are 54 contributors, 43 writing under their real full names or first names and nine writing under pseudonyms. The remaining two contributors have used both their real name and a pseudonym for different contributions, as they asked for some of their material to be anonymous. Coincidentally, several contributors share surnames despite not being related! In the text of *Living It Out* we have used first names only, or first name and initial for those contributors who share a first name.

Aidan Varney is a 27-year-old gay/queer man. Formerly Anglican, he is now a non-denominational Protestant.

Alex Huzzey is a 30-year-old gay man. A vicar's son, he is an Anglican with Open Evangelical leanings.

Annie Searle is a 34-year-old lesbian. Brought up within a Brethren community, she now worships at an Anglican church.

Anthony Searle is a 31-year-old gay man. Having experienced a broad spectrum of Anglicanism he has grown into high Anglo-Catholicism and he is currently training for ordination.

Bedford Earlobe is a bisexual man. Brought up middle-of-the-road Anglican, he has since become High Church Anglican.

Bill is a 55-year-old gay man and member of the Church of England.

Brenda Harrison is a 59-year-old lesbian and Evangelical Anglican.

Bruce is a 58-year-old straight man with a gay son. Previously a minister for the Assemblies of God, he now attends an Anglican church.

Charles Forman is a 25-year-old gay man and liberal Anglo-Catholic.

Chris Dicken is a 31-year-old gay man. His church background is New Church/Charismatic.

Christine Holt is 75 years old and a member of the Church of England. Her son is gay.

Daniel is a 30-year-old gay man. The son of missionaries, he grew up an Independent Evangelical and is now training to be a priest in the Anglican Church.

David is in his late 50s and a straight man with a gay son. His connection with the church started in Sunday school, he later became an Evangelical before 'developing an allergy to Evangelicalism'. He then spent six years as part of a Quaker Meeting before happily deciding to abstain from attendance totally.

Ed Arstall is a 51-year-old straight man. At the time of contributing a Baptist and new Christian of three years, he has since left his faith.

Elaine Ewart is a 33-year-old straight woman and member of the Church of England.

Guy Elsmore is a 42-year-old straight man. Ordained within the Church of England, he is currently Vicar of St Luke in the City Team Ministry in the centre of Liverpool, having previously been Area Dean of Widnes.

Gwilym Stone is a 25-year-old gay man and at the Anglo-Catholic end of the Church of England.

IP is a gay man.

James N is a 26-year-old gay man. Having grown up in the Charismatic Evangelical Church in the UK, he has since crossed the globe and is currently a member of the Uniting Church in Australia.

James Walker is a gay man.

Janet is a 55-year-old straight woman with a gay son. She worships at an Anglican church.

Jennifer C. Harding is a 44-year-old lesbian and Methodist.

Jeremy Marks is a 56-year-old gay man. In 1988 he founded (and still leads) Courage – initially an ex-gay organization, which became fully gay-affirming at the turn of the millennium. From an Anglican background initially, he has also been a member of a Baptist church and a house church.

Jim is a 24-year-old gay man in the Salvation Army.

Jo is a 42-year-old lesbian. Anglican by background, she places her spiritual home as with the Iona Community, recognizing their theology and expressions of worship.

John Simmonds is a 66-year-old straight man. A retired Methodist minister who has been heavily involved with championing LGB rights within Methodist structures, he is also involved in the Progressive Christianity network where people who feel at odds with traditional beliefs, structures and practices in churches find support, solace and challenge.

Karl is a 56-year-old gay man and Anglican.

Kate Rowley is a 22-year-old gay woman. She comes from an Evangelical Anglican background and now worships as part of the Metropolitan Community Church.

Leigh-Anne Stevenson is a 23-year-old lesbian and Baptist.

Lily is a 59-year-old straight woman with gay friends and a gay son. She is a member of the Church of England, where she is also a vicar's wife.

Margaret Evans is a 62-year-old straight woman. She has a

gay son and daughter, and works as a counsellor specializing in LGBT clients. Her interest arose because of 'the bishops behaving badly at Lambeth'. She describes herself as 'Anglican, sadly!'

Mark Burr is a 41-year-old straight man. His interest in LGB issues arose from a desire for the church to be characterized by acceptance, understanding and love. Baptist by baptism, he is an Evangelical Anglican in practice.

Martin Carr is a 31-year-old gay man and Anglican.

Michael Prior-Jones is a 27-year-old gay man. Mostly Church of England by background, he has also been involved in Methodist and Free Churches.

Naomi is a 28-year-old bisexual woman in a committed relationship with a woman. From an Evangelical background, she is currently a High Anglican.

Oscar is a 42-year-old gay man and Roman Catholic. He trained for six years to become a Jesuit priest but has since left and now works for a Catholic charity.

Paul Burgin is a 32-year-old straight man. His church background is Methodist/Anglican/Evangelical.

Paul Dicken is a 59-year-old father of a gay son. Founder of a Christian charity, he has been a committed Evangelical Christian for 43 years. He now describes himself as Evangelical in core doctrine but with reservations about negative values which lead to exclusion, intolerance, alienation and are contrary to Christ's love of all people.

Paul T is a 77-year-old homosexual and retired Roman Catholic parish priest.

Peter J. Crawford is a 25-year-old gay man. His church background is Methodist and Anglican.

Peter Hiscox is a 22-year-old gay man. From a Free Evangelical background, he is now a Quaker attender.

Reuben Walsh is a 16-year-old homosexual and Methodist.

Richard Hanson is a 25-year-old gay man and evangelist.

Richard Powell is a 30-year-old gay man. He describes his faith as 'a bit of a journey really', encompassing Evangelical, a bit of hyper-Charismatic, uber-Conservative Evangelical, Emerging Church, Anglo-Catholic and latterly no formal church but feels very much part of a 'Christian network'.

Rob is a 23-year-old gay man and Anglican.

Robert is a 51-year-old gay man and member of the Church of England.

Robyn Vesey is a 29-year-old straight woman, with a Church of England/ecumenical background.

Ruth is a 30-year-old lesbian, and (in her own words) 'moderate, dull C of E!'

Sally is a 36-year-old non-hetero and Christian.

Sarah B is a 32-year-old lesbian. Ordained in the Church of England, she is coming to the end of her curacy in a multi-cultural group of parishes.

Sarah Ingle is a lesbian. With a background in the Church of England, she has also attended a United Reformed church, and currently worships at a Methodist church.

Simon is a 21-year-old gay man. He describes his church background as 'complicated!' He did not grow up in the church, and attended an Anglican church from ages 16 to 19 followed by a Baptist church until 21. He recently started to attend a Quaker Meeting.

Sophie Manuel is a 25-year-old straight woman and a member of the Church of England.

Terry Biddington is a 51-year-old straight man. Ordained in the Anglican Church, he works as a university chaplain.

Tony Rablen is a 55-year-old straight man. Ordained in the Church of England, he currently works as a hospital chaplain and vicar's husband.

Vivien Holt is a 60-year-old heterosexual woman. She has a gay daughter and daughter-in-law.

Reaching for the rainbow: relating to God

Being gay is part of who I am, part of me. I cannot separate it or box it off or put a little fence around it so that it doesn't disturb the other aspects of me. I am a whole person in Christ, filled with grace and loved, as everyone is, by God. (Anthony)

We're starting at the heart of the issue. What's our faith about if it's not, at its heart, a relationship with God? It's that relationship that makes Christianity more than just a club, a comfort or a crutch. And it's the importance of that relationship, what it means at the core of who we are, that makes it impossible to ignore or shrug off controversy and challenge.

Realizing that you, a friend or a relative, are LGB can make you look hard at your relationship with God and ask the Creator a few tough questions. It means consciously choosing where you want to go with God, instead of just going with the flow. Many LGB Christians attribute their continuing, strengthened and enriched faith in God to the difficult path that they travel in reconciling their faith and sexual orientation. As friends or family of LGB people, you too may find your faith journey taking a different path from the one you first expected. Realizing that there are no simple choices or easy answers means working out, through laughter and tears, what really matters and celebrating what might otherwise be overlooked.

It's an opportunity, even if it's sometimes a painful one, for a new direction. Not everyone keeps their faith: many walk away from God or are put off even starting the journey. But forging a way forward is possible. Some find themselves in a new, deeper, more real place as they come to 'an understanding with God'. Some discover a journey outside current conventional Christianity that can be more Christlike, as well as more uncomfortable.

So in this chapter we explore how people are facing up to these dilemmas and continuing their relationship with God. We start with the reasons why some people leave God or church for a time, then hear advice about how we can keep learning about God and support each other in doing so, reflect on how listening to God can provide answers we seek – and end with the most important thing: love. Where are you on your journey? What can you learn from others who walk that road too?

Every path is different, but the experiences of leaving, learning, listening and loving which people have shared here may be familiar to you – or may help you to work out your next step.

Leaving

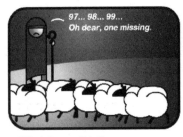 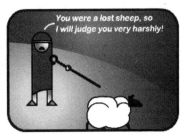

What Jesus didn't say.

There are countless different reasons why people leave their childhood faith, drop out of church or stop believing in God, but growing up as LGB or encountering LGB people and issues in a church environment can kick-start a questioning of values and assumptions. This may mean leaving church, it may even mean leaving God, whether for a short while, for years, for decades or for good. You may leave because you are made to feel that, because of your sexual orientation or that of a friend or family member, you cannot have a relationship with God. This is what happened to Richard H, who describes losing faith when he came out because he thought he had to. 'I thought faith and the gay lifestyle weren't compatible,' he explains, looking back. 'I thought that leaving my faith was what I was supposed to do, so I did, but then I came back into faith when I'd finally accepted my sexuality. I don't think I'd really accepted my sexuality until then.'

When asked which aspects of her faith were challenged by LGB issues, Sophie, who's straight, exclaims: 'Everything!' As she saw over and over again how the church responded to homosexuality and how Christians behaved towards her LGB friends, she started to question the fundamentals of her faith. It all came to a head 'one morning, at about 4a.m., after more than my share of booze. I suddenly thought, "If I have to choose between God and my friends, I'll choose my friends – what sort of a God is that?" Then I started thinking, "How do I know what God's like anyway?!" So that triggered a collapse of faith for me.'

As a teenager coming to terms with her sexual orientation, Leigh-Anne also felt that she faced a difficult choice. She reasoned that she couldn't be a lesbian and a Christian – at least that's the impression she got from talking to the youth pastor at her Baptist church – so she had to choose. 'One thing I knew, I didn't choose to be gay (like no one chooses to be straight) but I could choose to be a Christian,' she explains. 'If what my youth pastor said was right, it left me no choice but to give up my relationship with God.' But this wasn't an easy choice. 'This wasn't something I wanted to do; indeed I felt a loss, like my church and faith had been snatched away from me.'

Maybe you too will be familiar with this sense of disconnection between what you are told is right and what you yourself sense to be true. Especially as a teenager, surrounded by other pressures, this experience can make it extremely difficult to keep the faith. It can sound pretty bleak. But for some people, leaving (and returning) is freely chosen, not forced, a natural part of growing up. This was certainly true for Gwilym. Growing up in a family where 'you couldn't move for dog collars', he needed some time away as a teenager to find his own faith, but returned strengthened. 'Like many, straight and gay, the transition between the faith of my childhood and my adult faith involved a break,' he says. 'One didn't follow neatly on from the other – and during the gap of about five or so years in my teens, the realization and the reconciliation with being gay happened. So when I came back to faith at 16 or so, being gay was part of the person who came back.'

In describing this experience, Gwilym refers to the biblical story of Abraham's sacrifice of Isaac (Genesis 22), which showed him that 'we have to come to God willing to sacrifice anything. Everything is a gift from God, and in sacrificing it we are able to receive the gift afresh. There was a moment for me when accepting Jesus as Lord, and in doing that unconditionally, I had to sacrifice this aspect of my identity. While saying "this is who I am"; I said "but not my will but yours". I found a strong sense that I was being told to take hold of it again. In the wake of that experience of a vivid encounter with the embracing love of Christ, I have continued with a self-confidence in being a beloved gay child of God.'

The person who comes back will be different from the one who left. Coming out can be a catalyst for questioning, testing and challenging your whole faith and when this happens, take cover – the results can be far-reaching and explosive. When Peter H came out, his faith was already changing: 'I was starting to question elements of the faith I'd been brought up with. My church was splitting over how it was being led. The fact that the church was having difficulties and wasn't perfect stimulated me to think about what Christianity – and my faith – was all about,' he recalls. 'I had this routine of having to pray and read the Bible every day, then suddenly I thought "hang on, this is making no difference, and I can't see the point of it." I remember thinking "I can't keep putting this off for ever, I've got to think what this is all about and either make it work or stop it. I need a radical overhaul of my faith because it's not really working.'"

This radical overhaul not only brought him closer to God but allowed him to accept himself as gay for the first time. 'I'd already started to change the way I saw other things. It was certainly tied up together, questioning my sexuality and my faith at the same time. Without one there couldn't have been the other and I can see it now for the blessing that it is. The blessing of being gay has made me the person that I am now.'

Ruth was brought up as a liberal Anglican, and freely admits that she didn't have a big conversion or much of a personal faith. She went along to church because that's what you did. Only once she had drifted away from church after coming out, did she realize that her life was 'missing a grounding'. It might have been easier not to, but she chose to pick up her relationship with God again in adulthood. That's when the real work began. 'Then I had to try and integrate everything. That's still quite a battle even though I would say I'm quite happily a gay Christian. It's still a work in progress, I suppose it will be for the rest of my life.' Leaving – and returning – can be a necessary step. It helps you realize how important your faith is and allows you to own that faith for yourself.

While wandering in the wilderness, Moses received a call from God that changed his life (Exodus 3). Far from home, family and the certainties that had governed his life, he encountered God totally unexpectedly – well, who expects a talking bush? – and in a completely new way. Stories of such wilderness moments are scattered throughout the Bible. Jonah and Elijah are among those who, when their faith dipped so low that they were about to give up, went to the wilderness to rant and rave at God. We need those times away – scary and unsettling as they may be – to honestly face our difficulties and disappointments.

A crisis of faith or change of direction isn't necessarily connected with teenage angst. Bruce was an Assemblies of God minister with many years' experience of leading churches under his belt. Then his son came out. He started to question and re-evaluate his personal faith for the first time. 'For my wife

Janet and me, being able to identify with others of like mind has always been important,' he explains. 'Some of our happiest times were when we were totally committed to the work of our church, giving our all to its programmes and people. Having a gay son has forced us to stand alone. And when you do that in one area of your belief system, it frees you to question and look objectively at others as well.' Janet chips in: 'I've questioned my whole belief system in recent years. I've had doubts about my faith and the Bible. And I'm still very much on a journey. However, I believe God is in the middle of all of this.'

Their questioning led to big changes. Bruce left his job as a pastor and even though the couple now worship as part of an Anglican church, he doesn't believe they will ever fit into an organization again in the same way. 'Serving God wholeheartedly used to mean following your leaders wholeheartedly. Now it's more complex,' he says. 'We feel more responsible individually for our words and actions than before. It's far less cosy but we feel that the Lord is challenging us to be more mature and learn to love others just as much when we disagree with their doctrines as when we identify with them.'

Jo is not alone in only coming out – to herself, to God and to those around her – after many, many years spent living as a straight Christian. 'After coming out I had to come to terms with the fact that I'd been living a lie,' she says. This realization made her lose confidence in her own integrity and she still worries whether she or anyone else can trust herself, her words or her actions again. 'But, there is something about being broken, being flawed that is actually liberating,' she explains. 'I don't mean flawed because I'm gay, more flawed because I denied it for so long and hurt other people by pretending to be straight. It's liberating because it's a pretence that's broken, a false armour that felt like me but wasn't. I was inside. Now I have to learn to live without the false outer shell.' It was her relationship with God that finally helped her to break free and see herself for who she really was: 'I think I was out to God before I was out to myself. I think I told God years ago, when I wasn't listening, if you know what I mean. The gay me would pray when closet me wasn't paying attention. Eventually gay me got too loud for closet me to ignore – maybe God helped her to speak up! While I may feel exposed and vulnerable now, at least I'm not pretending any more.'

Leaving: Top Tips

- **Take a break.** You may have had it drilled into you not to leave God, and to always turn to God when times are tough. But maybe right now it's just too tough, the relationship's not working, and you need to take a break. God's not going to leave you, but is completely capable of holding you and your faith until you're ready to come back.
- **Expand your image of God.** How do you imagine God? Shepherd or lamb? King or servant? Mother or father? Fire or rain? Or what about a door, a potter or an eagle? These are all biblical images of God, but each gives us a different perspective on who God is. Think about whether some images have dominated your view of God at the expense of others. Maybe you need to leave some of these behind for now in order to see God afresh.

Learning

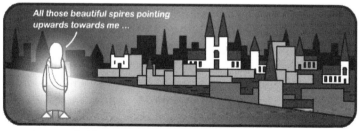

All those beautiful spires pointing upwards towards me ...

... when mostly I live over here.

Once you start challenging received wisdom and old certainties, that's when the questions really begin. It can seem that there's an impossible amount still to learn! The good news is that, although it may take time, there are lots of places to go for answers: books, prayer, support groups, a spiritual director or mentor, Bible-reading and, perhaps most importantly, learning from the people that God puts in our path.

Christine, now in her seventies, is a lifelong Christian. She says that she's read more scripture, more books about the Christian faith and taken a far greater interest in Anglican policy and politics since her son Adrian came out than ever before. She explains how shaken she was when she first realized how much she didn't know: 'During the years when our children had been attending church with us, joining fully in its life and worship – years, which to me as a parent had been so happy and fulfilling – unknown to us, Adrian had been growing in awareness that his developing sexuality was condemned by the church. Even though he had been at pains to conceal his feelings of same-sex attraction, it came as a great shock to me to realize that, even as his mother, I had not known anything about his inner turmoil; that I did not know our son as well as I had thought.'

So from a position of knowing nothing about LGB people or what the church had to say on the subject, Christine was driven to find answers to the difficult questions that her son's sexual orientation posed. She began to explore her faith through reading and conversation with others – and found that her relationship with God grew rather than weakened as a result: 'My faith in a loving and all-embracing God, as shown in the life and teaching of Jesus, has strengthened and deepened,' she says. 'I understand much more of Christ's teaching about love, gentleness, not judging people or causing them to stumble.'

When Jim, who like Christine's son grew up in church, was made to feel unwelcome in his Salvation Army corps because of being gay, he turned to his mum for support. She reminded him that it didn't matter what people thought of him, because his main relationship was with God and not with the church. This gave him strength and has stayed with him ever since. But it was not just her words that convinced him; he saw the truth lived out in her life. 'Now she's not able to get to a church

---

Spotlight on . . . rediscovering who God is

'I would ask straight Christians who God is for them. Whether God is the God who created the vastness of the whole wonderful universe and whose concern is for the entirety of humanity, and with enabling us to discover and respond to the injustices of the world and to the needs of our sisters and brothers across the globe. Or whether God is in fact vindictive, small-minded, crass, selfish and unloving, and prefers to be concerned with the relative insignificance of individual sexual orientation and with the intricate minutiae of how we find and express love and sexual pleasure.

'If straight Christians have any sympathy with the first view then it's high time we all stood up and said so.'

Terry

---

because of her disabilities and she's still going strong with her faith,' he explains. 'That experience gave me the strength to keep going.'

Bedford has found that returning to the age-old practices of worship, prayer and reading Scripture have helped him to feel accepted by God as a bisexual man. 'Despite all the times I've been told that my sexual preference "doesn't exist", or that I'm "going through a phase", or that it's "all about gay and straight",' he says, 'the problems have come from *other people* and I've still been able to look to God for refuge.'

Take heart, this is a time when you can learn new things about God, about yourself and about how to live your life. Whatever ways help you best to learn more of God, perhaps the most important thing is to keep on asking questions and not taking easy answers.

Learning: Top Tips

- **Search out other people's perspectives on their relationships with God.** It's not something we often discuss honestly, even in church! What are your burning questions? Ask some friends in a pub, at school, at work or in a church or Christian group.

- **Remember, you're not the only one.** You'll probably have realized already that it's not just LGB people who have to revisit and redefine their faith at least once in their lives (indeed, many of you will be straight people who are doing so right now). Some say that LGB people have an advantage, tending to get it over with earlier in life. So if you're LGB: remember your journey, it's something you could use one day as a gift to support others. If you're straight: why not talk to an LGB Christian? They may well have trodden this path before you.

- **Read widely.** Try the internet, and books from various publishers and authors. You may have been warned off some sources of information as 'unsound'. If you have tried to follow this advice for a long time and come to a dead end, now's your chance to rebel! Use the books you were warned off as an initial reading list. Look at the 'Where to go next' section at the back of this book. After all, God gave you a brain – so use it as you weigh up things you read.

- **Find a mentor or spiritual director.** This should be someone who knows the world well, who knows God well, who has heard it all before, and whose primary interest is to support you and your faith as it develops – not to control how he or she thinks it should develop. It may be someone from any section of the church. For example, Anglican dioceses have details of spiritual directors on their websites.

Listening

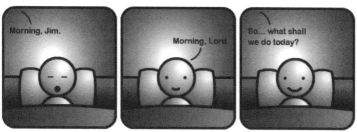

A perfect start to the day.

So you've been thinking, praying, talking, reading, wondering and worrying till you're worn through, but it still feels like you are going nowhere, unsure where to find God in it all. Time for another piece of practical wisdom from contributors to this book. But, be warned, it's tricky, at least it is for someone like me. I (Sarah) love to talk, and sometimes I only discover what I think after it comes out of my mouth, so listening to God, without jumping in with my own ideas first, is something I struggle with. I've never seen the clouds part or heard a voice come booming down, filling me with confidence that I've had a 'word' from God. I'm reassured to know that I'm not the only one who finds this hard, and that God is more likely to be heard as a 'still small voice' than a fanfare of trumpets. But building your own relationship with God may mean coming to a point where all you can do is stop – and try to listen to God, however scary that may seem.

Years had gone by since Leigh-Anne felt that she had to choose between being a lesbian and being a Christian, yet she felt she was still asking the same questions, still going over the same verses, round and round in circles. 'I was greatly frustrated that there was such a contrast in people's views,' she remembers. 'While the debate continued I was left in limbo as to whether or not I could be a Christian! But realizing that I hadn't got anywhere in five years made me realize that the church's view was never going to be unified in my lifetime. I couldn't wait that long to have a relationship with God.' So, what did she do? 'Instead of listening to people's views on the matter I decided for the first time to seek the only opinion that really mattered, God's!'

'In prayer I felt a question stir in me: "What do you feel?" What kind of question was that? Here I was desperately asking God the most important question of my life and he wanted to know how I felt?! And it dawned on me, all I felt was love, God's love. I had been so desperately asking God, "Is being gay a sin?" I had failed to recognize that I had never felt condemnation from God at all. What an idiot! To this day I am frustrated that I let the opinion of others define my relationship with God, especially as most, if not all, didn't even realize the impact it would have on my Christian faith.'

Yet despite the frustration and years of what felt like wasted time, Leigh-Anne now believes that good has come out of this: 'If it wasn't for this experience I wouldn't have been challenged to unravel my faith, to strip it right back to the bone and realize truly how much I love God. I often struggle, but my aim in life is to seek my happiness in God. So far I have felt only reassurance from God, my only condemnation has been from people who have pushed me away from God and church.'

Leigh-Anne is not unique among the people we've spoken to in having had an experience like this. Something remarkably similar happened to Chris. His background in a 'huge charismatic church, with big important leaders and big important things to do' meant that he was used to hearing messages from God confidently proclaimed Sunday after Sunday. But a focus on the 'big issues' like revival and salvation in church meant that he was left to his own devices when trying to hear God's word about his everyday life. No wonder he got impatient! 'One night I gave up with the Bible and tried talking to God directly,' he says. '"Come on!" I said, "You must have an opinion – you're God!" And actually, for one of the few times in my life, I got an answer.'

But, as Leigh-Anne found, when you look to God for an answer, you might get another question in return. Instead of condemnation, Chris heard the question 'What do *you* want?'

and being able to answer that question changed his whole attitude to being gay. 'I realized that it wasn't going to be about rules. It was about relationship,' says Chris now. 'If Jesus died to allow us to have a relationship with God, then surely me being gay is something I have to work out in that relationship. So I gave up with the black and white, and decided to live my life as a gay Christian man. I have given myself permission to make mistakes, and also decided never to lie about myself again. So all my Christian friends know I'm gay, and all my gay friends know I'm a Christian. God and I have an understanding I guess – I will try and live with honesty and integrity in a way that honours him and everything that he has done for me. And in return I ask that he lets me know if I'm doing anything that offends him. And so far it's worked out pretty well.'

Spotlight on . . . finding God on the margins

'One of the greatest fears that I have about people's relationships with God – and thus of my relationship with God – is complacency. There is of course the sin of not accepting God's love, but equally the sin of taking God's love for granted. Living a comfortable lifestyle in the UK breeds complacency in many aspects of life, so why not in religion as well?

'But God calls us not to rest inside our temples but to go out and "bring the good news to the poor". Not just as some act of altruism, but because it is with the poor, with the suffering, with those who mourn that we find God. The values of our society convince us that those in the centre are the ones with whom we should align ourselves. The values of the gospel call us to live at the margins.

'My admittedly small experience of campaigning for gay rights – Outrage's "Snog-in" at Piccadilly Circus, the gay equivalent of Gandhi's salt march – first made me aware of the much greater injustices in the world. And by seeing what it felt like to be on the margins I was better able to stand close to those who were even more marginalized – and there I would find God.'

Oscar

Listening: Top Tips

- **Listen to God.** This can seem very, very scary if you've been led to believe in a condemning God who will burn you up as soon as you consider a new thought. In our search for book contributors, we did not come across any stories of people hearing anything other than loving, kind and helpful things when they listened to God. This may have been when they were in the bath, in a busy meeting, or in a Bible study group. We did not hear of friends-of-friends who had been at the receiving end of a thunderbolt. So, get ready, take a deep breath, and risk it when you can.
- **Be honest about your failings as well as your feelings.** Are there things you regret that you have said or done in the past? Or activities or attitudes that you cling to which prevent you from having a relationship with God now? It's time to face these and ask for forgiveness. No matter how you feel, nothing is too big or too small for God's grace.

Loving

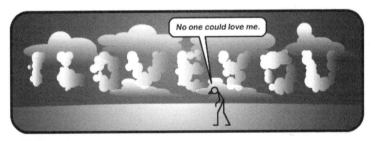

Think again.

Sophie has now found a way back to God, with the help of her parents: 'My mum said I don't have to be so angry, it's not my job. I then realized that I didn't have to carry the world's woes on my shoulders. That's what Jesus died for. Somehow that was a great relief.' She reminds us: 'If God made the universe,

God will stand up to a few questions no matter how scary it can feel.' We believe that a faith that asks questions, listens and learns, that has been through the wilderness and found its way home, can be a stronger faith, one that stretches without breaking.

All you need is love

'"Love the Lord your God with all your heart and with all your soul and with all your mind." This is the first and greatest com-mandment. And the second is like it: "Love your neighbour as yourself." All the Law and the Prophets hang on these two commandments.'

Jesus, Matthew 22.37–40

So what do we find when we reconnect with the heart of God? Jesus, St Paul and the Beatles all agree on the most import-ant thing – Love. Knowing that you are loved by God. Learn-ing to love yourself. Looking outward to love others. Here's how some of the contributors to this book have experienced and expressed that love. We'll close with their wisdom:

'After a long period of celibacy, emotional abstinence and spir-itual disconnection I decided in my forties to live my life no longer disregarding my preferred sexuality – women. I wanted to verbalize, put in writing and freely go to places that I could identify with, surrounded with people just like me – LGBT. I have to say: "Oh my God, I feel great!" God gave me free will; he loves me and because of this I've finally decided to live my life and no one else's.' (Jennifer)

'My faith was not really affected by having a gay child, for I believe that God made and loves each and every one of us, and therefore loves my child in the same way. I do not think of my child as "my LGB child" but as my child, and one thing about him is that he is gay – and I hope and pray that God feels the same!' (Lily)

'As gay people, we've often been through a lot – rejection, depression, or self-hatred. We may know what it's like to be lonely. That's why Christianity is, I believe, particularly for gay people. Jesus tells us he hasn't come to the rich, the successful, the centre. He has come to the edges. He has come for people like us, people like gay people. I've met so many gay people with a deep spiritual yearning and I really hope that we can respond to God's call. To share his vision of being acceptable just the way we are. To know that we are truly loved. To focus on building a better world.' (James N)

'What drew me to faith was the amazing, extravagant, outrageous, astonishing and incredible grace of God that says there's nothing I can do to make God love me more and nothing I can do to make God love me less. I take opportunities whenever they present themselves to challenge prejudice and bigotry towards the LGB community or any other people.' (Paul D)

'I find it sad that so many in the church are outraged by the appointment of openly gay people to roles of authority. What message do they give to the countless homosexual men and women who have turned away from God? That they are outsiders. Ironically, they thus become the very people that Jesus came to eat and drink with. Perhaps that is one reason why the Mass is so important to me. It is the place where Jesus loves me as me, and where I find the grace to live a more loving life.' (Sarah I)

A relationship with God is an adventure. It never stops changing, yet can always be relied on. It's unique and personal, yet connects us with the people around us. The following chapters get to grips with how we work out that relationship, at church, in school or close to home with family and friends – how we learn to live out the love of God.

Action

Draw a map of your own faith journey so far on a piece of paper. Mark the times you have especially known God's love and the people or experiences that have helped you on your way, as well as the wrong turns taken and time spent in the wilderness. Reflect on what this shows you about the past and what hope it gives you for the future.

Prayer

Take my life and let it be consecrated, Lord, to thee.
Take my moments and my days, let them flow in ceaseless
  praise.
Take my struggles, take my fears,
Guide me through the coming years.
Take my life, all I've been through,
Use it, Lord, to draw near you.
Amen

(adapted from words of the hymn by Frances Ridley Havergal)

The good book?

I grew up in an Evangelical Christian home, where the Bible was supposedly the sole authority on all questions of life and faith. (Daniel)

The Brethren movement always emphasized that it is everyone's right to read and to interpret the Bible. Perhaps this independence paradoxically gave me confidence in my unorthodox views. (Annie)

As a Roman Catholic, I have never felt that biblical texts can be used to support or condemn homosexuality. My problem has been more with church teaching. (Paul T)

One really nice thing about charismatic churches is no one really talks about the Bible that much. (Chris)

Four people, four traditions, four different views of the Bible. You may have heard, from Christians and non-Christians alike, that the Bible is 'perfectly clear on the issue of homosexuality'. But with such divergent views on the importance and status of the Bible, can this really be the case?

We both came to faith in self-proclaimed 'Bible believing' churches with conservative approaches to the Bible. The kind of churches that have posters outside promoting 'God's instruction manual' and where a sermon shorter than 40 minutes is a rare event. It was some time into each of our Christian journeys before we understood that it's possible to have a Christian faith that doesn't centre on a literal reading of the Bible. We've found that being LGB and Christian has meant having to spend time rereading and rethinking our understandings of the Bible. It's brought us into contact with people from different denominations and backgrounds, helping us to discover more creative and inclusive approaches to the biblical texts. We have learnt that taking the Bible seriously is not the same as taking it literally.

However, having such a Bible-focused upbringing gave me (Sarah) a valuable gift: the 'memory verse'. As a child in Sunday school, I learnt chunks of Scripture off by heart, from single verses to entire psalms, and these Bible passages remain with me still. Words of encouragement, hope and mystery have become part of me, understood in new ways as I've grown older, familiar and fresh at the same time. In this chapter, we have encouraged people to share their own 'memory verses', the words that have inspired them and that they return to again and again.

We'll also be sharing some of their insights and experiences that come from reading the 'good book' from an LGB perspective. These range from advice to take a break from the Bible altogether, to encouragement to tackle difficult passages head on. The latter part of the chapter suggests ways in which we can bring today's questions to the Bible: by going back to first principles, putting what we read into context, and by reading in relationship with God and with fellow believers. We hope this gives a flavour of ways in which people have got to grips with the beautiful, dangerous, holy, disturbing, comforting and sometimes downright bizarre set of texts found in the Bible.

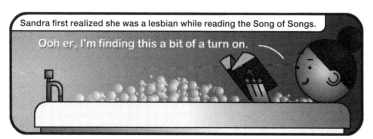

Just one more person set free by the beauty of Scripture.

Take a break

But, before you read any further, stop right here. Is there a sinking feeling in your stomach? Have you had so many bad experiences of the Bible that even thinking about it makes you feel sick? Is this chapter like a mouth ulcer – you'd rather it wasn't there or that you could forget about it, but can't stop yourself from coming back? You don't have to read on – we'd much rather you gave yourself a break.

At a retreat a few years ago, we met a young lesbian trying to figure out how to find God, after a decade or so of abuse at the hands of her parents and church as they had tried to force her to be straight. She couldn't stop clinging to her Bible, and reading Philippians over and over again. When asked why, she explained that it was the only book in the whole Bible that didn't contain any passages that someone had used to condemn her, and she was still looking for the promised Good News. That week, she found more of God in reading the lesbian magazine *Diva*, and discussion and prayer with a wise lesbian nun.

So, if you've wrestled for years with the Bible or if it's been used as a weapon against you, if even thinking about the Bible brings you out in a cold sweat – stop. You do not *have* to read it. Do not fear (as the biblical authors repeatedly tell us). Here are a few tried and tested alternatives:

'Look around for alternatives to the Bible, preferably unfamiliar ones, because you won't react with aversion to these, and will find yourself stimulated by the difference of thought pattern. For example, I use the Apocrypha occasionally in private worship. Beyond that, there are plenty of other books or novels written by Christians or about the Christian message, some of which are very refreshing. Try Julian of Norwich for starters; she portrays our relationship with God in such positive and caring terms.' (David)

'I used to read the Bible every day at university, but I rarely pick it up these days unless I'm really upset or wondering about a

Memory verse: Revelation 21.1–4

'Then I saw a new heaven and a new earth, for the first heaven and the first earth had passed away, and there was no longer any sea. I saw the Holy City, the new Jerusalem, coming down out of heaven from God, prepared as a bride beautifully dressed for her husband. And I heard a loud voice from the throne saying, "Now the dwelling of God is among people, and he will live with them. They will be his people, and God himself will be with them and be their God. He will wipe every tear from their eyes. There will be no more death or mourning or crying or pain, for the old order of things has passed away."'

'During Lent one year I spent several weeks being upset and feeling alone at the church I was going to. I felt sure that everyone would hate me if I came out to them. But suddenly and unexpectedly I came across these words from the book of Revelation, set to music by Bainton. As I sang them I had an overpowering feeling. It was as if God was telling me that he made me as I am and that he not only loves me, but likes me. I knew then that the period of my life when I had struggled to accept myself as a gay Christian was over. With Easter would come a new start with fresh hope. I realized that even though many Christians would react against me as a gay man, I would have the strength to carry on fighting, knowing this love for me.'

Charles

particular issue. Then I tend to pick up a Bible, open it at random and see what it says. I believe God has the grace to show me something useful at those times.' (Sophie)

'I do think that there is a danger in relying entirely on the Bible – God does speak to us in other ways, and often these experiences feed back into our reading of the Bible. For people who find reading the Bible anxiety-inducing rather than helpful, it might be time to look elsewhere for the Good News – sometimes a talk with a friend, a film, a walk in the country or a good novel can bring you just as close to God.' (Elaine)

'I find my spiritual input in people and places, in poetry and pilgrimage (even if only virtual), which I need to keep me sane and to keep my horizons widened.' (Lily)

Memory verse: Psalm 139.14–16

'I praise you because I am fearfully and wonderfully made; your works are wonderful, I know that full well. My frame was not hidden from you when I was made in the secret place. When I was woven together in the depths of the earth, your eyes saw my unformed body. All the days ordained for me were written in your book before one of them came to be.'

'I'm still unclear about some aspects of homosexuality that I haven't got my head round yet, but I am utterly convinced that God's heart is open to all people. God knew that some of us would be born disabled, some black, some gay, some lesbian and some white, heterosexual or able-bodied. Every one of us is equally precious, and equally loved by God.'

Paul D

Face the clobber texts

The way that the Bible is used has an impact on *all* of us, whatever kind of Christianity we personally identify with. Interpretations of passages in both Old and New Testaments which have been used to exclude and condemn LGB people risk being seen as the only legitimate ones. These passages (Leviticus 18.22 and Romans 1.21, 26–27 being best known) are sometimes called the 'clobber texts'. Interpretations of these texts that show LGB people as disordered, intrinsically sinful or misguided have turned many of us away from the Bible, from the church or from God, and prevented countless others from considering that Christianity may have something to offer to their lives. We heard a teenage girl speak up at a Christian conference we attended recently. She explained how she had invited her non-Christian friends to a youth service at her church, but said they were put off returning after hearing a church leader condemn gay people by saying that verses in Genesis showed that 'God created Adam and Eve, not Adam and Steve'. Even when cited without any harm intended, clobber verses and their interpretations have made many people, straight or LGB, feel unwelcome.

Maybe you've read these verses in so many different translations that you are now not sure what to make of them. Maybe they just don't fit with your experience of God. Maybe you believe the interpretations that show that it isn't possible to be LGB and a Christian, but find this too painful to bear. There are plenty of books and websites which question the legitimacy of these interpretations of the well-worn clobber texts (see the 'Where to go next' section at the back of this book). So if you come from a tradition that warns you against dismissing these texts – or even makes them central to your understanding of Christianity – then these resources are worth exploring. Taking time to pray, read, think and tackle them head on may be a vital part of your journey.

Memory verse: Galatians 4.27

'For it is written: "Be glad, O barren woman, who bears no children; break forth and cry aloud, you who have no labour pains; because more are the children of the desolate woman than of her who has a husband."'

'God's gracious inclusion of the social and sexual outsider is overwhelming and unexpected. Reading and rereading Galatians, I experienced God's parental love as a warm embrace, as if I was being held in God's arms.'

Daniel

Robyn describes herself as a 'straight friend, who feels that any kind of prejudice and discrimination is wrong' and her firm views on the clobber texts help set a framework in which we can begin to re-examine them: 'I don't think God wants us to clobber each other with Scripture or with anything else!' she says. 'When I read the Bible I understand Scripture in the light of my faith in an inclusive God. I like the idea of being able to feel protest and rebellion against God, and against Scripture too, to ask God – WHY did you put those bits in when they have been used in a way that causes pain?'

Bringing today's questions to the Bible

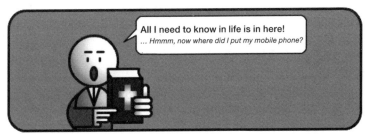

So ... it isn't then.

'It's the challenge of every era to come back to Jesus' words anew and figure out what the big principles mean for our lives every day,' says James N. As his faith has developed, the debate about specific verses which can preoccupy evangelical Christians no longer interests him. Instead he's passionate about bringing the principles and the stories found in the Bible alive to address the burning issues being debated today, in the church, on newspaper letters' pages and radio talkshows.

Instead of expecting answers direct from the pages of the Bible, James suggests looking there for ideas that will help us resolve today's big questions for ourselves. One example he gives is found in Acts 15, which describes 'a big discussion and heaps of controversy over whether or not gentiles should get circumcised, or what they could eat. To everyone's relief, they decided that they could keep their willies intact, and they could still put prawns on the BBQ. To us, these disagreements seem stupid and irrelevant. But what issues are splitting the church today?' James asks. 'There is one big one – is it OK to be gay? Does loving and serving one another mean it's OK to be gay or lesbian? How do we know what's right? Well, there's a lot about how we make that decision if you look in the Bible.'

Back to basics

So, instead of providing neat answers to every question, the Bible can help us to work out our own answers by reminding us of what's most important about our faith.

It took Bruce some time to see the Bible in this way. He started out his Christian life convinced that the Bible condemned homosexuality – and a good many other things too. 'I became a Christian at 18 and joined a fundamentalist church,' he explains. 'We believed we were the one true church and that we must observe every command in the Bible. So we kept the Saturday Sabbath, wouldn't eat pork or seafood and paid triple tithes. It was easy to understand the Bible at that time. "God said it, I believe it and that settles it!" was our mantra.' As an Assemblies of God pastor, he taught his congregation – and his five children – to strictly follow the Scriptures. But he now realizes that, even before he discovered that his middle son was gay, this view was slowly shifting. 'I think that God was preparing me because, one by one, I began to see that many legalistic beliefs that I had held over the years were wrong. I was becoming more liberal in my outlook by degrees, but this certainly didn't extend to believing that you could be gay and a Christian in good standing.'

When his son came out, Bruce went back to first principles and set to studying again, but it wasn't an easy or comfortable process: 'Starting to see the Bible differently on issues such as a Saturday Sabbath sprung a huge leak in my particular boat, but coming to understand the truth about gays holed me below the waterline. My whole doctrinal supertanker sank. There

> **Memory verse: John 15.18**
>
> *'If the world hates you, keep in mind that it hated me first.'*
>
> 'For me personally, even as I've been hurt and rejected by my parents, my Christian friends were always there for me when it was tough. There's always a place for gay and lesbian people within church, because they often need community more than most. Furthermore, for every gay and lesbian person who feels rejected and judged by society as immoral – so was Jesus! He was an outcast and was even crucified for supposedly breaking religious law.'
>
> **James N**

was a real danger of spiritual shipwreck at this time, because it would have been so easy to throw everything out of the window and say, "The Bible isn't the infallible word of God, it's only people's ideas and some of them are just plain wrong."'

For Bruce, as for many others, the internet was invaluable and he read many books. As a result of experience, study, reflection and by the grace of God, he has now come to the belief that 'we have fundamentally been interpreting the Scriptures wrongly. We have taken proof texts and used them to support our own ideas and then bash others over the head with them. We have imagined that the Bible is internally consistent in its theology as if it were written as a manual for living, when in fact it is neither. It is God's word for us but we need to understand in what way. We need to interpret both the Old and New Testaments in the light of God's law of love.'

Simon has also needed to find new ways of approaching the Bible. Still in his early twenties, his experiences as a gay man have prompted him to think about how the Bible is interpreted, and in particular, about how formerly mainstream interpretations on other issues have since shifted or been revised. 'I find it very difficult to accept the Bible as entirely the literal word of God,' he says. 'I have difficulty with a six-day creation, apparent endorsements of slavery and other issues. I also feel driven away from the Bible because it has been used to try to condemn my homosexuality and limit me to a life of singleness and repressing my deepest feelings.' Despite this, he still believes that the Bible is divine: 'The simple principles "Do justly, love mercy and walk humbly with God" and "Love God, and love your neighbour as yourself" have tremendous power. I have found much wisdom in the Bible.'

Spotlight on . . . a bisexual view of the Bible

'One thing I find infuriating about "The Big Gay Debate" is that it is argued in black and white terms: gay and straight. We are told by one side that we must all be straight, and we are told by the other side that we must be accepting of gays. It is rare that the bisexual perspective gets a look-in! When the gay liberation theologians tell us that our forefather David must have been a homosexual because he loved Saul's son Jonathan "as his own soul" they frequently forget to tell us that he also had no less than eight wives and assorted concubines, not to mention that he successfully fathered copious babies with them . . . Such matters are, it would seem, irrelevant, if David being gay proves a point – and he is not the only bisexual this has happened to: Oscar Wilde and Sappho are just two of history's hijacked bisexuals ("bijacked" might be an appropriate term).'

Bedford

Putting it in context

The realization that the Bible no longer seems 'perfectly clear' can be shocking and unsettling, but shouldn't stop us using it to help guide the decisions we make about how to live our lives. It doesn't automatically mean a life of hesitancy and provisos. Instead, difficult verses can start to make more sense when put into historical context and embraced as part of the bigger picture the Bible gives of God's overwhelming love for all.

Engaging with this bigger picture means no longer unquestioningly accepting each verse as if it came straight from the mouth of God as reported by your favourite church leader. This can be a huge challenge for those of us, like John, who grew up with the idea of the Bible as the cornerstone of our faith and the complete, infallible and unchanging word of God. But it can also open up new, creative and enriching approaches to the biblical texts.

'Until I was 25, I was a conservative evangelical – someone who gave equal value to every word of the Bible as the "inspired Word of God"' explains John, a retired Methodist minister. 'Then it dawned, slowly at first, then with revolutionary force, that Bible writers were each coloured by their own experiences and conditioned by their own communities and culture. It also dawned on me that those who have studied, commented upon and preached from sacred Scripture down the ages have likewise been conditioned by personal, cultural and community aspirations. The Bible ceased to be a fixed and absolute authority and became a kaleidoscope of human engagement with the mystery of God and the circumstances of the day.'

How does such a radical change of view take place? Jeremy has led an ex-gay organization which, based on a traditional evangelical understanding of the Bible, encouraged and supported LGB people to remain celibate. He helps us shed light on an answer. 'Very rarely does one change one's understanding of Scripture without a strong external imperative to do so,' he says. The external imperative came for him when he realized over many years that his organization's approach was not working. 'I receive enquiries, especially from the media, that ask, "What day did you decide you had to change your approach?" assuming that there must have been some blinding moment of revelation, a Damascus Road type of experience, but it did not happen like that,' he continues. 'The Damascus Road story sounds more interesting. Nobody likes to think that realization dawns gradually through a long winter, while

---

Memory verse: Genesis 18.10–15

'Then the Lord said, "I will surely return to you about this time next year, and Sarah your wife will have a son."

'Now Sarah was listening at the entrance to the tent, which was behind him. Abraham and Sarah were already old and well advanced in years, and Sarah was past the age of childbearing. So Sarah laughed to herself as she thought, "After I am worn out and my master is old, will I now have this pleasure?"

'Then the Lord said to Abraham, "Why did Sarah laugh and say, 'Will I really have a child, now that I am old?' Is anything too hard for the Lord? I will return to you at the appointed time next year and Sarah will have a son."

'Sarah was afraid, so she lied and said, "I did not laugh."

'But he said, "Yes, you did laugh."'

'I think one of the things the Bible shares with us is that God has a sense of humour – the habit of asking unlikely people to do impossible tasks is in part a playful habit. We shouldn't be ashamed, like Sarah was, to laugh at God. I often find myself saying "You must be joking, Lord!" And the answer is usually, "Well, yes, but I still want you to do it." For gay Christians there are perhaps more "you must be joking" moments and a greater awareness of the possibility of holy laughter – but this is a good thing, it acts as a defence against being self-righteous and also gives us a way to keep going when we have the "if I didn't laugh I would cry" feeling.'

Gwilym

---

just plodding on through life.' As he changed his views, Jeremy began to turn the organization around, but was left wondering how to make sense of Scriptures that he had never doubted prohibited homosexuality in any context – loving or not.

He eventually realized that 'none of the Scriptures written by Moses or Paul, that have for so long been used to outlaw and exclude gay people, were ever intended by their human authors or by God to give pastoral guidance on the care of lesbian and gay Christians. On the contrary, the clobber passages are in fact addressing godlessness, idolatry and the use, exploitation and abuse of others for selfish ends. At long last I came to see the real peril of deception, that comes from blindly pursuing so-called biblical principles instead of learning from the truth.' So where is truth to be found? Jeremy answers very simply: 'Jesus Christ.'

Reading in relationship

When we read the Bible we do not do so in isolation, but from within a relationship with God and as part of a community of believers: those around us today, those whose stories are told in its pages and those who have read and interpreted it throughout history. We read it in the light of these relationships and in order to learn how to live in relationship with others. Relationships are never easy, so this is maybe why we so often struggle and disagree about how to relate to the Bible.

When Chris, whose words head this chapter, searched the Bible for answers about whether it was OK to be LGB and a Christian, he didn't find them. Instead he found the Bible to be complicated and contradictory, reflecting the complexities of humankind's relationship with God. Yet there were still principles and examples that could help him in his own relationships. 'The relationships we have as human beings are never neat and straightforward, and our relationships with God over the years clearly haven't been any different,' he reflects. 'So I didn't get the clear answers I was looking for from studying the Bible, but what I did learn was something about what's important to God and what isn't important. What is clearly important in the area of relationships is that God's into faithfulness, honouring one another, and being honest.'

As Chris discovered, the way in which we interpret the Bible can have a lasting impact on how we understand relationships, for good or for ill. Daniel, who is also quoted at the start of this chapter, found that the understanding of the Bible that he

Memory verse: Acts 10.9–23

'About noon the following day as they were on their journey and approaching the city, Peter went up on the roof to pray. He became hungry and wanted something to eat, and while the meal was being prepared, he fell into a trance. He saw heaven opened and something like a large sheet being let down to earth by its four corners. It contained all kinds of four-footed animals, as well as reptiles of the earth and birds of the air. Then a voice told him, "Get up, Peter. Kill and eat."

'"Surely not, Lord!" Peter replied. "I have never eaten anything impure or unclean."

'The voice spoke to him a second time, "Do not call anything impure that God has made clean." This happened three times, and immediately the sheet was taken back to heaven.

'While Peter was wondering about the meaning of the vision, the men sent by Cornelius found out where Simon's house was and stopped at the gate. They called out, asking if Simon who was known as Peter was staying there.

'While Peter was still thinking about the vision, the Spirit said to him, "Simon, three men are looking for you. So get up and go downstairs. Do not hesitate to go with them, for I have sent them." Peter went down and said to the men, "I'm the one you're looking for. Why have you come?"

'The men replied, "We have come from Cornelius the centurion. He is a righteous and God-fearing man, who is respected by all the Jewish people. A holy angel told him to have you come to his house so that he could hear what you have to say." Then Peter invited the men into the house to be his guests.'

'One time I was feeling a bit perplexed as I had some really good Christian friends who are lesbians and I wasn't really sure what I thought. I went to sit on some grass between their house and mine, and opened the Bible. I think I might have even prayed a bit for guidance first! This passage appeared and at that point I felt reassured that it was all good. I felt very much that God was calling my friends "clean".'

Sophie

was brought up with damaged his ability to form relationships with the people around him. It dominated his imagination and dictated his views on the nature of God and the immorality of his emerging sexual desires. 'I grew up with a closed mind,' he says. 'I genuinely believed that same-sex desire was "detestable" and that God would punish me for it. I allowed this way of thinking to limit my development both spiritually and emotionally for too many years, hiding my sexual desire in perfectionism, academic achievement and Christian work. When I finally came out to friends and family, I had to dismantle my understanding of God and the Bible piece by piece – a painful process from which I still have a lot of residual anger.'

Yet, his story doesn't end there: 'The process of coming out was a spiritual and intellectual liberation, helping me to engage my mind and imagination as well as my body and my emotions. I have now ended up with a larger, richer and more awe-inspiring view of God, and a fresher, more exciting approach to Scripture. I thank God for this work of the Spirit in my life.'

Martin, whose love for the Bible inspired him to enrol on a biblical studies master's course at the age of 31, believes that it has much to say about sexuality, but only in the broader context of relationship. 'The question the Bible really asks is how do we relate to one another and to God, irrespective of who we are. The characters of the Bible aren't so different to us really. They knew God in their lives. Through their stories in the pages of the Bible, I believe we too, whether gay or straight, can be touched by the love of God,' he explains. 'There is no naivety in the Bible about sexuality, which, with its potential both for good and for evil, forms part of the motivation that guides human action. The Bible tells us stories, of David and Jonathan, of Jacob and Rachel, of Ruth and Naomi, of David and Bathsheba, of Jesus and the beloved disciple, not to give us rules of sexual behaviour, but to instruct us in human loyalty and compassion, and the destructive consequences when selfish desire and the lust for power take control. It is not the "who" of relationship that matters to the Bible, indeed it can

Memory verse: John 8.3–11

'The teachers of the law and the Pharisees brought in a woman caught in adultery. They made her stand before the group and said to Jesus, "Teacher, this woman was caught in the act of adultery. In the Law Moses commanded us to stone such women. Now what do you say?" They were using this question as a trap, in order to have a basis for accusing him.

'But Jesus bent down and started to write on the ground with his finger. When they kept on questioning him, he straightened up and said to them, "If any one of you is without sin, let him be the first to throw a stone at her." Again he stooped down and wrote on the ground.

'At this, those who heard began to go away one at a time, the older ones first, until only Jesus was left, with the woman still standing there. Jesus straightened up and asked her, "Woman, where are they? Has no one condemned you?"

'"No one, sir," she said.

'"Then neither do I condemn you," Jesus declared. "Go now and leave your life of sin."'

'The story of the woman taken in adultery is used by both sides of this sort of argument. One side says "Look, Jesus didn't condemn her" and the other side says "Yes, but he told her to sin no more." The detail I find interesting is Jesus writing in the sand. We go on and on about sex, either for or against. It is so easy to latch on to it as an area where actions are unambiguous. Some think (with good reason) that sex is dangerous and must be controlled. Some think it is to be celebrated and enjoyed (which may often be appropriate). Both sides think it is unavoidable and of overwhelming importance. But Jesus just goes on writing. Perhaps he is bored by the whole subject of sex, as opposed to relationships.'

Bill

be man and woman, rich and poor, Jew and Samaritan, sinner and righteous person, but the "how" of that relationship that matters.'

Like Martin, we find it deeply frustrating that so much of the discussion about sexuality to date has concerned the 'who' not 'how' of relationship. Time and energy is taken up debating whether same-sex relationships are permissible, with both sides using Bible verses to prove a point or support what they already believe to be the case. But there is little serious discussion about how strong, godly, lasting relationships – between people of the same gender or of different genders – can be nurtured and supported using biblical models. Unless we let the Bible speak into our relationships, and the realities of our lives, Jeremy says, 'The Christian life is just about studying a book to get the "right" understanding of Instructions-To-Be-Obeyed, rather than having a relationship with the living God who dwells among us, drawing us to himself.'

Memory verse: Hosea 2.23b

'I will say to those called "Not my people", "You are my people"; and they will say, "You are my God."'

'God calls all of us. God loves all of us. Gay people today are seen as unholy, unclean, just like, say, lepers or foreigners in Jesus' time. When Jesus breaks down the barriers, everyone, including gay and lesbian people, are invited to participate. This is such a beautiful prophecy. All of us, including gay people, are invited to join God's banquet. None of us can be turned away.'

James N

What the Bible really says

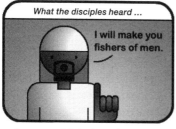 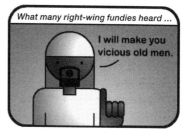

An easy mistake to make.

As biblical scholars, poets and dreamers, we can all arm our-selves with determination to strip away age-old prejudice and read the Bible afresh, not as a rule book, but as a book of empowerment, hope, love and reconciliation. There may be side effects – you might feel dizzy, confused or overwhelmed at first – especially when trying to put to one side what society, to say nothing of the church, tells us the Bible says. James N again:

'It sometimes seems that the only time we hear about the Bible is when it is used to justify conservative values. Somehow the Bible is used to support the message that stresses working hard and making money, being law-abiding, having a family and kids, not drinking and so on. It's so ironic then that, at its heart, through the story and person of Jesus, what Chris-tianity revolves around is so radical. We find out that contrary to conservatives, Jesus didn't work hard – instead he left his job, and called others to leave theirs, or at least stop aspects of their jobs that were exploiting others. Jesus didn't marry or have kids and he repeatedly ignored his own parents. Jesus drank alcohol. He broke the law, repeatedly, and was finally killed for it.

'Jesus didn't conform. His life and teachings are the exact opposite of what so many Christians tell us "the Bible says". People say they follow Jesus but so often they seem to live the opposite to how he lived and say things that are opposite to what he said. A lot of Christians never really engage with the

Memory verse: 1 Peter 2.7

'Now to you who believe, this stone is precious. But to those who do not believe, "The stone the builders rejected has become the capstone."'

'I was moved by a sermon in the Abbey on Iona on this text. As I reflected on the inclusive ministry of Jesus – and the experience of Jesus himself – it seemed to me that I could no longer discriminate. I needed even to support the cause of those rejected: I joined the Lesbian and Gay Christian Movement.'

Tony

Jesus story, never really look to it for guidance for their own lives.'

If you come to conclusions about what the Bible has to say about LGB people, about Jesus and about how to live your life following God, that are different from the ones held by your church, your friends or your family, you might be accused of being a selective Bible reader, only choosing the texts you agree with and not accepting the Truth. This accusation often comes from people who say they would love to be more accepting of LGB people, then sigh, shake their heads and say 'But the Bible says . . .' Take it from us, you are not the only selective Bible reader. It's the nature of reading such a complex book, and every Christian does it whether or not they are aware of doing so.

'The Bible contains six admonishments to homosexuals and 362 admonishments to heterosexuals. That doesn't mean that God doesn't love heterosexuals. It's just that they need more supervision.'

Lynn Lavner, US comedian

Whatever viewpoints we hold, we will all encounter people at some point who hold different biblical interpretations from our own. Simon has advice that everyone would do well to follow in this situation: 'Never accuse people of being soft-hearted if they don't wish to follow your interpretation of the Bible,' he says. 'The odds are they'll still value support. Try to understand everybody's point of view, and accept that others may think differently.'

Yet even after you have come to terms with the Bible for yourself, and particularly the clobber texts, you may still find yourself sitting through sermons or Bible studies, dreading the day that one of Those Verses comes up. We'll give the last word to Leigh-Anne. When she started in a new church and a new home-group, she decided to be honest with people whom she hoped she could trust, making an effort to drop things in conversation that would make it obvious she was a lesbian. Yet this fear still remained. 'In my home-group we happened to study one of the gay-bashing verses,' she recalls. 'This is it, I thought, here's where I get battered and have to leave this church. So I decided to sit through it without saying anything. But to my surprise people acknowledged that the verse had done much harm to the gay community and that it was today totally taken out of context. Wow, fantastic! I'm sure that their view doesn't reflect the whole church but just knowing that there are people who share my views is a great strength.'

Action

'Being "biblical" actually means going against the grain, taking a stand for what is right and just, and daring to believe that God may see the world in entirely the opposite way to how most people imagine it. This view of the Bible is entirely consonant with how Jesus handled Scripture: "You have heard that it was said . . . but I tell you . . ."' (Terry)

Is there a verse or passage in the Bible that particularly troubles you? Read it and then take it to Jesus. Imagine him saying, 'You

37

have heard that it was said . . . but I tell you . . . ' about this passage and see if you can hear what new thing God is saying to help you understand these difficult words afresh.

Prayer

Author of our lives, you call each of us to play our part in the Bible's story, to meet its challenge and challenge it in turn. Forgive us when we try to misuse or control it. Show us its power to transform us and touch us through its pages with your love. Amen.

(from words by Martin)

3

Should I stay or should I go?

> Those of us who have been touched by Jesus and know his love find ourselves misunderstood by the gay and lesbian community for continuing to stay in the church, and also know ourselves to be misunderstood by the church for being who we are. Perhaps we are therefore those who are most greatly blessed. It often feels so to me. (Sarah I)

Imagine the scene if all the LGB people, their friends and families, left the church tomorrow: the empty pulpits, the missing musicians, the people in hospital left unvisited and no one to teach the Sunday school! Let's face it, the church relies on us. Yet sometimes it is just too hard to stay in church because we are made to feel that our views and experiences are unwelcome.

When people talk – and when we write here – about church, it's normally to refer to a particular local church. But (inter)national policies influence local churches and, conversely, the experience of belonging to the wider, worldwide body of believers is a fundamental part of being a Christian. Staying in – or leaving – church can be simply a matter of changing what you do on a Sunday, or be as far-reaching as whether you continue to identify as a Christian.

When I (Rachel) first came out, I could see that there were *some* LGB Christians in the church, but only among male High Anglican clergy. How did a young, lesbian evangelical like myself fit in? A decade on, I have discovered a wider range of role models and I'm still hanging on in there in church. So, if you are struggling to see how your church background, beliefs or worship style can possibly fit with your understanding of LGB issues, read on.

Church *can* be a positive experience for LGB people, their families and allies. Yes, it's true! Churches that provide a warm welcome are not restricted to any one denomination or style. You may not always find them in lists of LGB-affirming places of worship (see 'Where to go next' at the back of this book) or read anything overt in their literature, but they do exist. That's the case with the local Methodist church where we now worship. It's a small church, with a good mix of people, who have welcomed us warmly. Our sexual orientation is a non-issue there. Maybe there's a church like this just around the corner from you.

But, that said, virtually every person who contributed to this book has spoken of failed attempts to fit in and painful experiences of rejection before they found a place to believe and belong. Some have still not found that place and have given up looking, or have friends who have rejected the church after being rejected themselves. The good news is that there are ways we can stay in churches while keeping faith and integrity. But how can we negotiate the potential trauma without damaging ourselves or others in the church? What are some of the signs that it's time to leave – or that it's time to stay for good? We'll be sharing the stories of those who decided to leave a particular church in search of somewhere more inclusive, those who have stayed in the church despite the challenges they've faced and those who have left church or found a spiritual home elsewhere.

You should go! (. . . somewhere else)

Sarah I, whose words head this chapter, is a dangerous person to have in your church. At least that was the pastoral assistant's view at the United Reformed church where she worshipped some ten years ago. 'When I told her I wanted to say something about being a lesbian in a church meeting on the "Human Sexuality" debate, her first words were "Oh no! You'll split the church,"' Sarah recalls. 'However, I knew I was not on my

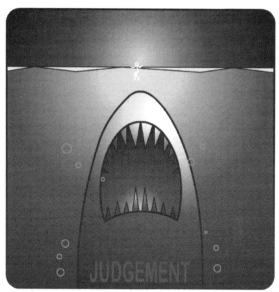

Just when you thought it was safe to go back into church ...

own: there were others like me within the URC, which gave me the confidence to ignore that comment and to speak out.'

Although she was listened to politely on that occasion – and the church didn't split as a result – Sarah became wary about expressing herself. Then a new minister arrived who believed that LGB people were in need of healing. Not one to give up easily, she had a long meeting with him, one to one, at the end of which he conceded that it was possible that 'a few, a very few, gays and lesbians might be born that way'. 'However, I was so uncomfortable receiving communion from someone with the basic belief that I was not acceptable as I was,' says Sarah, 'that I wrote a letter to the elders and left the church. I spent the next two years wandering in a lonely wilderness, unwilling to risk rejection again.'

Eventually, she found the courage to return to church, this time to an Anglican church recommended by a lesbian friend. It was an emotional homecoming: 'The first time I went, my friends were not there, but as the congregation began to sing the Gloria, I started to weep. I had so missed a worshipping community. I had never before worshipped with icons and incense, and so many candles, but I loved it and was transformed by the caring community there, so much so that I found the courage to enter a loving, intimate lesbian relationship which has brought me great peace and happiness.'

Rebuilding trust, even after only one or two negative experiences, takes a long time. After leaving a church that we had been attending but where we felt sidelined and eventually pushed out, paranoia set in. After that, every time we went to any church service, we expected someone to condemn our relationship from the pulpit, give us dirty looks during communion or choke on their after-church coffee when we introduced ourselves as a couple. This didn't happen, but 'just because I'm paranoid doesn't mean they're not out to get me', in the words of the old joke, seemed to be an entirely reasonable position to hold for some time. We still find it creeping up on us now.

Leaving home to study, having children, getting older, moving house or finding a partner are all reasons why people move from one church to another. Life changes, and what we look for in a church changes too. Faith develops along new paths; different needs and different ways to serve arise. Difficulties around sexual orientation are only one reason for leaving a church – but long-held hurts can make it difficult to take the plunge again. The messages that come from some public Christian voices don't necessarily help either! This doesn't surprise Peter C. He's still a churchgoer, but sees why many of his friends have replaced Sunday morning worship with a Sunday morning lie-in. 'Nominally Christian friends tell me that the only voice of Christianity reaching them on the streets emphasizes a need for repentance, rather than encouraging them to worship,' he says. 'Add to this the public image, and previous experience, of the church as homophobic, and I can fully appreciate why people expect a church experience to be an uncomfortable one of condemnation.'

An uncomfortable experience of condemnation? We can't see that ever becoming a strapline on an Alpha course poster. It wouldn't tempt us to get out of bed on a Sunday either. But church doesn't have to be that way, as Simon has found. He tried several different churches during his teens and early twenties, but often felt isolated, wondering how he would be thought of and treated if people knew that he was gay: 'I have also been told many times, directly and through literature and other media, that I have to fight and completely repress my homosexuality to be a Christian. This is unhelpful when I believe the opposite and accept being gay. It can make me feel like I am failing God even when I don't believe that I am.' But finding the Quakers gave him the opportunity to explore his faith in a new way: 'I can focus on what matters to me, without hearing the repeated suggestions, that secular people never do any real good and Christians are better, that used to drive me nuts in my previous churches. I've made new friends and have been able to learn more about how to live my life in a peaceful, caring, and simple way.'

Annie's sexual orientation also prompted her to move away from the denominational background of her childhood. 'I grew up in first a Brethren Meeting, then an evangelical free church. There was no discussion of sexuality in the former and much hyperbolic and emotive discussion in the latter,' she says. She has now made her spiritual home in the Anglican Church, even though there is much she still values about her Nonconformist upbringing. 'I miss the commitment people have to their free church, as well as the extensive Bible knowledge the Brethren members have, but I appreciate the more open-minded, inclusive attitude of the Anglican churches I've been in. In each, my partner and I have been accepted (rather than tolerated). In fact, in our first church together, we were fêted!'

Elaine has also experienced very different kinds of churches. She grew up in 'a middle-of-the-road Anglican church which was far too polite to talk about sexual matters from the pulpit', so it wasn't until university that she came across churches which were specific about anti-LGB views, as well as proclaiming that women should submit to men in marriage, and that those who didn't believe in Jesus were going to hell. She explains why, as a straight woman, she deliberately sought out a more inclusive church instead: 'To me these were all issues of justice. As well as my church background, I had just as strong a background in liberal secular society that seeks to value all human beings equally. So eventually I moved to a more liberal church. In some ways, it was more liberal than I was entirely comfortable with at the time, but it seemed the most honest place for me to be. In this way, LGB issues shaped my approach to issues of faith, even before I knew any openly LGB people at all well. Now I can say that I have been humbled as well as enriched in my Christian journey by the stories of gay friends and acquaintances whose lives, either as single people or as couples, have been examples of Christian faith – sometimes within the church, sometimes outside it – and of tolerance, honesty and love.'

We have found, as Annie, Simon and Elaine did, that worshipping in churches with different styles, theologies and denominational labels can be eye-opening and inspiring. It's an opportunity to realize that the church of God is more diverse and dynamic, contradictory and confusing than you ever expected it to be. Jesus' prayer that his followers would be one, just as he and his Father are one, might tempt us to believe that 'being one' means everyone being the same (which means, of course, everyone agreeing with me). Instead, perhaps it is about learning to see the spark of God within the differences and discovering that there are different ways to express the same faith, that enable many people to stay in church.

Naomi, a self-defined church outsider who has tried all sorts of churches from the very charismatic through to Anglo-Catholic, puts it like this: 'I've tried to leave the church on numerous occasions and couldn't. God has said, "No, you're not going to." I've always felt a huge outsider in the church for loads of reasons, gay being one of them, but also specific learning difficulties, mental health problems, other problems. Every time I went to a church, especially between the ages of 18 and 20, I would feel really uncomfortable. And I dealt one at a time with the things that were causing me grief about the church, and slowly realized that actually nobody's perfect, and

---

Spotlight on . . . how one church has shut LGB people and their friends out

'Tammy was one of my best friends. Kind, warm, helpful, and someone who I came to love as if she were a sister. She was also someone who was at the fringes of church life feeling that, because she was gay, she wasn't welcome. It didn't help when we were both at a church service and the curate calmly criticized homosexual practice. Each sentence he uttered felt like a wound, so how it felt for Tammy I cannot imagine. She did not want to go to another service and I felt that in one evening, my hard work in trying to show a positive side to Christianity, where Tammy would feel at home, had been undone. She died following an accident four years ago, and I wish I could have told her that her friendship and thoughtfulness – whether it was dropping everything to help me stand for the local District Council elections to advising me on, well, anything really – made me wake up and want to see a better attitude from various sections of the church towards the gay community.'

Paul B

---

you can't find a church that's going to be. God tells me where he wants me to be when. There are always things to learn, new ways to think. I feel quite privileged.'

Top Tips: How do you know it's time to go?

There are sometimes good reasons for leaving a church. It may feel like giving up, even when leaving is the bravest and most difficult course of action, but it does not make you a failure. Here is some advice from people who have faced that decision.

- 'Listen to your instincts. Don't force yourself to stay if all you want to do is run out of the door!' (Sophie)

- 'The moment to go is when the struggle of staying becomes so big that it excludes the opportunity to experience God. And when you go, I think the advice of Jesus when he sent out the disciples is useful – in towns where they weren't welcomed he tells them to kick the dust from their feet as they leave (Matthew 10.14). I think that's about leaving the whole situation behind and not taking the bitterness of rejection with you. The dust and the dirt of that broken relationship should not be carried with you to pollute new places.' (Gwilym)
- 'Following the example of Jesus, the church is meant to be a place where people can "discover how to flourish" (John 10.10). If your church, its people or clergy prevent you from doing this or from believing that you're in every way the equal of everybody else, then it's high time you found somewhere else.' (Terry)

You should stay! (. . . if you can)

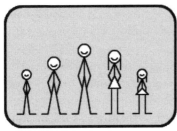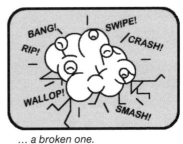

The church is a family ...   ... a broken one.

Leigh-Anne struggled to find an accepting church for many years, until stumbling upon a Methodist church in a nearby village. Cautious about getting involved if it meant facing rejection again, she emailed the pastor up front. In her email, she explained that she was a lesbian and wanted to attend a church where she could focus on growing her relationship with God, rather than worrying about being condemned. The answer was positive but she still wasn't sure: 'The pastor was great, saying this wouldn't be a problem. Although I was very dubious at first about whether this was really true, I went along. During months of sitting on the edge of my seat during sermons and home-group waiting for the "God hates gays and wants you to change" speeches that I get so paranoid about, I slowly realized that they really weren't going to come. Hooray!'

Although you might not believe it from reading the papers, sexual orientation isn't the only issue ever discussed and dealt with in church. As Leigh-Anne found, most members of churches have more pressing things to worry about than who fancies whom. So churches with a positive, inclusive attitude to all different types of people, especially those marginalized by society, can be welcoming places for LGB people, their friends and families, whether or not they make this explicit. They are nourishing places because they understand and accept people as they are. This is the kind of church that Alex grew up in and believes provided a great basis for remaining fairly level-headed about being LGB and being a Christian. It's also the kind of church that left its mark on him and that he still seeks out as an adult.

'Even though most people in the congregation would have thought gay relationships were wrong for Christians, it was a church where people were very real and honest,' he explains. 'Everyone knew that life didn't always work out the way you thought it was supposed to. Depression, divorce, bereavement and mental illness were part of lots of people's stories, and people knew that none of that made you any less a Christian or any less a member of the church family.' Watching people go up and down to the communion rail in that church is still a very moving experience for Alex. It reminds him that being LGB is only one of many things in people's lives that some churches have got upset about over the years, and used to stigmatize their members. 'I'm still not sure what most of them think about the gay issue,' he says now, 'but they're a constant reminder that being part of a church is less about thinking the right thing about every issue, and much more about being part of a family of believers.'

A sense of belonging to that 'family of believers' has not come easy for James N. He grew up in what he describes as 'a fairly conservative church'. Maybe that's a bit of an under-statement: 'My mum used to do ex-gay counselling for the church, before she gave up through lack of success,' he says. 'I'd always believed that being gay is wrong, but as a teenager I realized that I liked guys not girls. I stopped going to church for a long time because I just couldn't deal with it. I couldn't reconcile who I was with what I believed about homosexuality. I couldn't reconcile the God of love and acceptance that Jesus talked about with the God they preached about in church.'

Yet now he is passionate about encouraging others not to give up. 'I know a number of gay Christians who don't go to church, who have given up on church,' he says. 'They feel they have been rejected by church as I was and so they rejected it in return. If you feel this way, I want to urge you: don't give up. If you don't believe in hierarchy, Jesus didn't believe in hierarchy either. But he did believe in community. Because we funda-mentally express our faith in the way we relate to each other, I don't think it's really possible to be a Christian alone. We may need to go through that time apart from the Christian commu-nity, but at some point we have to come out of the wilderness. We need to share together, comfort each other, help each other. As Christians, following Jesus isn't about what we can get, it's about what we have to give. Just like he did, we are called to give everything for each other.

'I think churches need to be challenged, straight Christians need to have gay friends. It's a lot harder to hate gay people when you have gay friends. We need to be there, doing our best to live out God's dream. We need to be a witness in the church to Jesus' inclusive vision. Because I think that the only way people's attitudes are going to change is when the other – gay people – become one of them. One of us. So don't give up on church, don't give up on God, because he hasn't given up on you.'

Sally was strongly rooted in the Baptist Church, having been a member for nearly 20 years. During this time she married and divorced and got on with the business of bringing up her daughter as a lone parent. But a few years ago she began to quietly come to terms with herself as a lesbian who was open to the possibility of finding a partner. She did not want to give up on church, but realized that the culture of silence regarding the relationship between her faith and her sexual orientation was tearing her apart. Finally it was a heated discussion on sexuality in her house-group that made Sally realize that she had to make a stand. When a discussion about the acceptability of cohabitation – for heterosexual couples – moved on to same-sex couples, she found herself a lone voice in maintaining that sexual orientation of whatever type is a gift from God to be used responsibly. Around her she heard comments like, 'Homosexuals won't get into heaven', 'Gay people need healing', 'It's like alcoholism', and 'The church has to make a stand somewhere.'

At home that evening she began a long process of thinking and praying. 'I realized that, according to what I'd heard at housegroup, if I found a partner I wouldn't be welcome in the church on an equal basis,' she explains. 'If I were, it would cause other people pain and possibly cause them to leave. That was something I wasn't about to have on my conscience. So I prayed about it and thought about it and prayed about it some more. Then I formulated my letter of resignation from church membership.'

But her involvement with the church didn't end there. While Sally's letter stated blandly that due to differences on one issue she didn't feel it was appropriate to remain a church member, she did explain her intention to remain an active part of the congregation. Aware that some people would want to know why she had resigned her membership, she told them privately before it was announced at the church members' meeting. 'At that point something amazing started to happen,' recalls Sally. 'Faced with somebody coming out whose faith they knew, people started to think about the issue again and reassess what they had said. My friend, who had claimed homosexuals wouldn't get into heaven, apologized because she realized

Spotlight on . . . how one church is welcoming LGB people and their friends in

'St Luke's is a wonderful neo-classical building, but over the years, the congregation and the community lost touch with one another and numbers declined. In 2005, there were just five in the congregation, but we had a clear sense that God hadn't finished with St Luke's and that we were being called to something new. Throughout 2006, a careful analysis of our strengths and of the area's needs produced a plan for renewing and relaunching the church. In November that year, we made a new beginning. Six months on, the response has been tremendous, we now regularly have up to 40 worshippers across two Sunday services and have found a new sense of mission and calling. There is a large gay community in the parish and the congregation felt strongly that welcoming gay parishioners and affirming their God-given sexuality was a step we wanted to take in a very public and joyful way. Offering prayer with those joined in civil partnership in the same way that we offer weddings, baptisms and funerals to the parish and striving to make our worship LGBT-inclusive has helped us to broaden our vision of what it means to be a community, of who God is and of how God welcomes all of us.'

Guy, Vicar of St Luke in the City Team Ministry

what she had said was probably wrong and must have hurt me. It doesn't mean we have a totally similar understanding of the issues but we have started to move into dialogue. A number of my friends in church now think more about the impact of their words and how they form their opinions. When my resignation was announced to the church meeting they were careful not to out me, although I think it was probably pretty obvious where my differences with the dominant thinking in the church lay.'

So what changed in her local church as a result of her action? 'I know if the same discussion happened now there would be less ignorance and more sensitivity; more actual thought would go into people's responses. On a personal level, I was just as fully included being out as I was when I lived in the closet: occasionally helping out with Sunday school, joining the catering team for cafe church and doing the church chairs. It was business as usual and I think that it would have been the same if I had a partner. Being honest and breaking the culture of silence in the church in a way which still treated the majority view with respect worked.'

Despite not sharing the majority view, Sally was able to stay in her church, maintain her integrity and gently challenge other people to re-evaluate their beliefs. This is a cause for celebration but very difficult balance to strike, and not one that is right for everyone.

Top Tips: Finding a church to stay in

In some churches, staying can be difficult. It may mean being excluded from certain activities or making painful compromises. Many stay because of family and friends, loyalty to the church or enthusiasm for style of worship or activities. Or they stay, as Ruth has, because it's a core part of their faith. She explains: 'As Christians I think we are meant to bear witness to our faith in community. But as LGB people, our slightly disjointed relationship with many Christian communities affects our personal faith. I guess I would say that I'm Christian in spite of the church and not because of it. In some ways that has given me a greater depth of faith. Every time I go to church and feel uneasy, I have to ask myself why I'm staying and I think that does constantly make me re-evaluate my faith and why it is important.'

There are suggestions in the next chapter, 'Coming out in church', to help churches to become places where LGB people, their friends and families want to stay. But we'd also like to share some tried and tested strategies to use whether you're on a church-search or wondering if it's worth sticking with the one you're in.

- **Take your time:** 'Choosing a church is difficult, it's a difficult grouping to get under the skin of – always presenting a "nice" face to the world and patting itself on the back about how welcoming it is. It takes time to really get to know what it's like.' (Lily)
- **Don't go asking for trouble:** 'Find a church that at least does not take a hard line against homo- and bi-sexuality. The majority of churchgoing should be a positive experience, rather than one that regularly troubles you. Being LGB is *important*, and yet a *part* of who a person is.' (Peter C)
- **Look local:** 'I think that attending my local church is the best option for me. However, if it causes you to suffer spiritually (a terrible thing to say about your local church, I know, but it can!) then it's better to withdraw and ask the Lord to give you support elsewhere.' (Bruce)
- **It's not a perfect family:** 'Church is a family, and a dysfunctional one. I have yet to meet a functional family. They all have their arguments and quarrels, but the most successful ones keep talking and talk honestly.' (Anthony)
- **Set an example:** 'I know personally I couldn't deal with having to challenge other people, because I have to look after myself and protect myself as well. But the most powerful thing I've found is when people can show an example so that others realize that LGB people are not like such and such from the television.' (Charles)
- **Seek it out:** 'God is creating a new family, graciously transforming and rearranging nature. Nowhere is this kind of family more in evidence than in a church or Christian community that accepts and nourishes people of all backgrounds, ages and sexual orientations. I would encourage anyone, whether LGB or not, to seek out such a community, or if possible to work towards the transformation of the community in which you find yourself.' (Daniel)
- **Pray about it:** 'If you come to a conclusion that you feel gives you integrity but also works for the greatest good, it's likely you've become aware of God's will.' (Sally)

You should go! (. . . God's outside too)

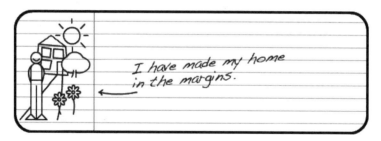

I have made my home
in the margins.

While Sally made her stand by resigning church membership but staying within the church, Margaret, whose son and daughter have both come out, felt she had to leave the church in order to keep her integrity.

'With the bishops' talk of potential schism, I have created my own schism with the Anglican Church,' she says, explaining the difficult process that brought her to this decision. 'I do not wish to attend or be part of a homophobic, prejudiced, ignorant church, while maintaining my profession as an affirming, accepting and non-judgemental counsellor. I teeter uncomfortably on the edge – unable to fully let go, nor yet to come in again. It is not a secure or comfortable place, but it is where I have been for a number of years, unable to move.' She feels uneasy with this decision: 'I do feel guilty for not attending any more. I have had leadership positions in the past and so am well placed to challenge people's opinions, but I just do not have the emotional strength to do it.

'Only two or three people in my local church have noticed that I am not there any more and have commented. I was obviously not as important as I thought. One of these kind ladies always talks encouragingly to me as I come to ring the bells, and she hopes I will come back. But I do not want to be pitied or looked at as an outsider who needs a special invitation to come to church. Jesus welcomed all – but if my children or other representatives in the homosexual population are not welcome there and the church makes different rules for gay clergy, then I do not belong there.'

Margaret's 'schism with the church' was a vital, if person-ally difficult, way for her to take back control, to say enough to injustice, exclusion and discrimination. Such attitudes had no place in her professional life or personal faith. Aidan, a gay man in his twenties who used to attend a high-profile evangeli-cal church, had a similar realization and response. 'There were lots of people who disagreed with me in the church,' he says now, 'but for a long time I didn't say anything. In the end that wasn't enough – I was too political. One day in the bookshop I found a book about healing gay people, and thought I can't be in this place, this is just nonsense, I don't need healing.'

Witnessing the experiences of her LGB Christian friends has forced Robyn as a straight woman to think afresh about her church engagement. As a result, she's forged a faith indepen-dent from, but she hopes still in relationship with, the church. After moving towns a couple of years ago she hasn't started going to church again. Why? 'I still find it difficult to walk into new churches, worrying "will I be safe here or will I be judged?" It's mostly the church hierarchy rather than God that I worry about, but vicars and priests are authority figures and, although I don't like to admit it, their attitude and evalu-ation of me somehow matters. Particularly attitudes towards these deeply personal and vulnerable parts of ourselves like sexuality.'

Peter H has also found it hard to settle in a church: 'It's not just being gay, it's the unspoken expectation that you must believe a certain thing or behave a certain way,' he says, articulating a feeling that causes many people in their teens and twenties to drift away from church. 'I've found that hard because I want to be in a church where I feel I can be com-pletely myself at all times, where I can say "actually I don't know what I think about Jesus and sometimes the whole Jesus thing confuses me". But there seem to be unspoken questions that you can't ask and topics that you can't discuss, of which being gay is always one.'

But how could church be different? 'I think that church ideally needs to facilitate the individual's journey and needs to have that open space for people to say when they don't agree with what's taught. But too often churches become like institutions that are just trying to protect themselves, making other people believe what they want us to believe,' Peter continues.

While churches stand to lose if they don't listen to these voices, the risk for LGB people and their allies is equally if not more significant. It's the risk of becoming so dragged down and bitter about 'what the Church has done to me' as to stop seeing ourselves as part of the church at all, to become permanent outsiders.

But it doesn't have to be this way. 'The idea of inside/outside the church doesn't really make sense to me as so much of my family and social life is made up of interactions with Christians,' explains Gwilym, who has found strength in a more fluid model of church. 'For me, "the church" doesn't really have an outside. Support comes from these networks which transcend the local congregation that I am a part of. Any rejection that might occur in a local expression of the church would have no power to change my sense of belonging, as that belonging is founded in the bigger network.'

Many of us share that sense of belonging to something bigger, whether we have been rejected many times or welcomed with open arms, whether we've decided to stay in or to go from a local congregation. We don't need to fight to get into the church, we are already part of it. This chapter throws out a challenge to all of us still in the institutional church – how can we learn to be more honest about our questions, difficulties and differences? Changing the church begins right here with each one of us, with you, with me.

Action

Reflect on the people and places that make up 'church' for you at the moment. It might be the community you worship with on a Sunday, being part of a group of friends who talk and eat together, a feeling of belonging during a Christian event or connections made in an internet forum. Thank God for what you value most about the relationships with these people.

Prayer

Spirit of God, you move like the wind, disturbing us, refreshing us, always taking us onwards. Forgive us when we are reluctant to follow you to new places or fail to notice how you are breathing new life into familiar ones. Wherever we are, however we worship, thank you for calling each one of us to be part of your people. Amen.

4

Coming out in church

I don't feel troubled by the fact that some people in the church probably disapprove of our relationship; the church has a number of divorcees and single mums, for example, and no one voices disapproval. For a congregation consisting principally of well-heeled *Daily Telegraph* readers, I feel this is rather remarkable. (Annie)

Coming out can be described as if it is a once-in-a-lifetime event, the single dramatic moment when it's revealed that Clark Kent, whom everyone thought they knew so well, isn't just a mild-mannered reporter, but likes to wear tights and save the world from disaster in his spare time.

Yet, in our experience, coming out – about your own sexual orientation, or that of a friend or relative – isn't a one-off experience. You are likely to have to come out and out and out again. In some settings you'll still be Clark and in others simply Superman. Church can be one of the places where you remain in the closet for longest, even once your family, friends and workplace are all in the know.

Since being a couple, we've always been out when attending church together. It's felt the easiest approach, otherwise there are so many questions to avoid and so much explaining to do. We feel that dishonesty, even if only by omission, would get in the way of building genuine relationships within the church family. This approach has entailed meetings with ministers (you'll find our top tips later), and had its moments of horror, relief, comedy and anticlimax. It has also brought its own difficulties: people are sometimes unable to see beyond the fact that we are in a lesbian relationship, while we can have a tendency to put up a front as 'super-Christians' in order to prove to people that we are Christians at all.

At times it has also been surprisingly difficult to convince people that we really are a couple! New acquaintances tend to start off assuming we are flatmates, then that we're sisters (perhaps because they see we share a bond closer than friendship), before finally accepting with great puzzlement that we are actually married (only once we've shown them all the wedding photos and our civil partnership certificate in triplicate). Perhaps it's because existing stereotypes about 'the homosexual lifestyle' are so strong. One of our friends told us that until he actually met LGB people, his understanding came entirely from media reports of cottaging and pictures of Pride marches. LGB people weren't like the people he knew and he certainly never saw LGB Christians portrayed.

So, why might you want to share the news? How can you tell when the time is right? As Rob straightforwardly puts it: 'Before you come out, you believe that it's all going to go wrong.' But is that what always happens? Although you don't need to be a super-hero to cope, it is best to be prepared. We hope this chapter – including a handy 'Coming out in church checklist' at the end – will give you some of the information, courage and confidence that you need, whether you are thinking about coming out in church yourself, wondering how open to be about an LGB relative, or are a minister wanting to support LGB people and their families in your congregation.

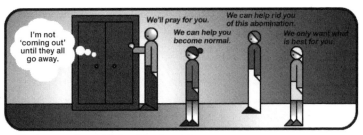

Maybe sometimes it's best to stay put.

Coming out over coffee

We've found that it has been simpler to come out in church as a couple. Not only because we can support each other if it all goes pear-shaped, but because people understand more easily about relationships than about orientations. Gwilym explains how awkward coming out can be for single LGB people in church: 'There's a difference if it is a natural thing, having a partner and going to church together; that's part of your life. But if you're single it becomes a slightly odd thing to start talking about. You can't easily discuss it over coffee.' Despite this he does remember some occasions where 'coming out has simply been a case of flirting over a glass of sherry after Mass!'

Peter H had been attending his church for some time, and only decided to come out there once he started a new relationship. He wanted to be confident that, if he brought his boyfriend to church, they would both receive a warm welcome. But soon he discovered an even more fundamental reason for coming out: 'It's not just "would they still accept me now I was in a relationship?"' he concludes. 'It's "do they accept me for who I am?" That isn't dependent on whether I'm in a relationship or not.'

Bedford wonders how some people in his church might respond if they knew he was bisexual: 'Would they be comfortable with a bisexual in their midst? Would they group the bisexuals in with the gays? And if they did, would it be with hostile intention?' Usually he gets round this by not mentioning his sexual orientation since, understandably enough, 'when talking to the elderly ladies pouring the teas I see no reason to discuss my sex life at all'. For him, as for many of us – straight or LGB – it's only when after-church chat turns to genuine friendship, that sharing more intimate parts of life becomes appropriate. As Bedford says, 'The church people with whom I am comfortable discussing my sexuality are, more often than not, people with whom I have developed enough of a rapport to discuss such matters as I would with my other friends.'

Once you start forming these genuine relationships with

others in church, then the closet can start to close in. Jennifer came out in midlife after finding the constraints of years of secrecy too much to bear. Things reached crisis point, with suicidal feelings dominating her experience of church: 'The long hard journey of being in the closet was emotionally exhausting,' she says, looking back. 'I swung from Jekyll to Hyde on a daily basis and struggled to keep up the pretence as I became older. At times I felt suicidal, clearly because I wasn't living my life. I wasn't being me. Even though part of me was dying daily, I initially convinced myself that it would be wrong to come out.' When she eventually did start coming out, Jennifer felt a burden had lifted and found that the consequences of doing so were not nearly as bad as she had feared.

For Christine, as for many other people with an LGB family member, coming out has become a natural – and thankfully positive – part of everyday life. 'Having a photograph of my son Adrian and his partner, taken at their blessing ceremony, alongside one of our daughter and her husband taken on their wedding day, has helped to start many an interesting conversation,' she says. 'Our experience of coming out at church has been a very gradual process, and yet very liberating. We have met largely with acceptance and understanding.'

I (Rachel) can vouch for this, having found that coming out can help deepen relationships in church. For a while (longer than was wise!) we attended a church that really struggled with our relationship, as we really struggled with how they responded to us. After a few months of keeping quiet about how hard we were finding it, I started to let people know. Suddenly, I found myself in genuine conversations over coffee – the older woman who didn't feel she could tell anyone in church that her son was in prison; the vicar's daughter negotiating her private and very public life. We are still in touch with people from that church, with deep friendships even several years after leaving it.

While it can be difficult for LGB people to come out in church, it can also be difficult to be on the receiving end of the news, whatever your views. 'If you come out to a relative stranger in a way that puts them on the spot, they may say the wrong thing out of sheer nervousness,' Elaine explains. 'There are probably just as many well-meaning folk with foot-in-mouth syndrome as there are mindless bigots. More, hopefully.' Paul D encountered the 'foot-in-mouth syndrome' once he started to come out in church about his gay son: 'One or two individuals in the church were unaware of Chris's sexuality, and made shallow and uninformed statements about homosexuals. When I quietly told them that my son is gay, they fell over themselves to backtrack and say that they personally had no problem.'

Coming out, as the term suggests, makes you vulnerable. It's the act of stepping out from the shadows, apart from the crowd or away from other people's expectations and showing a deep part of yourself to another person. It can happen even very late in life, maybe motivated by a desire for someone other than God to know about a previously secret part of you. During a discussion about LGB issues at a Christian arts festival, I (Rachel) was part of a small group which included an 83-year-old woman. She told me with a knowing gaze: 'My husband died two years ago after 60 years together. We'd always been so happy. I've never told anyone this, but I do wonder, if I'd been young now, if my life would have been different.' I felt privileged to have been the first person she had come out to, and I often wonder whether afterwards she was content never to come out to anyone else or whether this was just the start of a whole new direction in her life.

After all, as Peter H learnt, sexual orientation is not just about our relationships, it's about who we are in ourselves. The God we worship together in church is the same God who created, knows and loves these unique parts of ourselves. One of the hardest but most fundamental challenges we face is to see, accept and embrace the uniqueness of the person in the next pew as they were created to be, not as we might want them to be, and to accept our own uniqueness too. The labels of 'liberal', 'evangelical' or 'traditional' that we give ourselves and others, and that are sometimes used as shorthand for whether or not we affirm same-sex relationships, can stand in the way – as Mark, a straight man and active member of a large evangelical church, has found. After hearing a sermon on 'listening to the gay community' and getting to know LGB Christians, his 'traditional evangelical' position shifted towards an acceptance of long-term same-sex relationships. He now has his own coming out to do: 'I have experienced a faint echo of what being gay in church might be like in being labelled as a "liberal",' he says. 'I wonder how my existing evangelical friends will react when I "come out".'

Worry about the implications for her ministry has prevented Sarah B, an Anglican curate, from coming out to many people at the church where she works. Some of her colleagues and parishioners know or have guessed her sexual orientation, but most are unaware. She describes what a fine and difficult balance this can be: 'I have had to find language which I can use to describe my partner to parishioners without either coming out to them or feeling like I'm denying our relationship. When she is visiting, we avoid using any descriptive nouns. I don't use "friend", because that does not distinguish her from my other platonic friends. On the other hand, "partner" is too explicit. Normally I say, "This is Diana. She is a priest from the States. We met when I was at divinity school over there." My heart sinks when I say it, because my heart and eyes are telling me how much I love her and how the person standing next to me is going to be my wife.'

Coming out to the 'experts'

When you, or a friend or family member, first come out, you may not know what to think. You may want to hear the church's view from a trusted minister or youth leader, to get answers to questions or find guidance at a confusing or distressing time.

We know from the previous chapters that Leigh-Anne is now confident in her sexual orientation and has found a welcoming and accepting church, but she did not find it an easy journey to reach that point. As a teenager, she was very involved in her church: joining in Bible studies, playing in the band and becoming a church member. Yet she had no idea what the church's views on being LGB were – it had simply never been discussed. Reassured by finding LGB-friendly resources while surfing the net, she resolved to speak to the church's youth pastor about her findings and feelings. Leigh-Anne consulted him, but 'unfortunately, he wasn't as convinced as I was on what I had found, and simply offered that I was still "welcome" at the church (too bloody right, I had been there all my life!) and told me that "God loved the sinner not the sin".' With those words now in her mind, she began to feel uncomfortable at church, wondering if she was sinning. So uncomfortable that she stopped taking part in activities and eventually left the church: 'I felt that I wasn't worthy to even set foot in church,' she says. 'So I decided to take a break to figure it out.'

Also in his teens, Alex plucked up the courage to go to a seminar at a Christian conference on 'the gay issue'. He listened carefully as the speakers told anecdotes about LGB people they had known who were mostly sad, confused, mixed-up individuals, and as they ruled out any suggestion that a same-sex relationship could ever be satisfying or mutually fulfilling. They talked about demons: not all LGB people had a demon, they admitted, but some almost certainly did, and just needed delivering. They referred to a male vicar, who was living with his male partner. 'I hate to say it,' said the speaker, 'but that man is not saved.'

At the end of the seminar Alex queued up to talk to the speaker. Over a decade later, he still remembers how he felt that night: 'My heart was thumping. "I think I might be gay, and was wondering if you could point me in the direction of some people who might be able to help me." "How old are you? 18? Don't be silly, you'll grow out of that." That evening I was in bits. A very precious secret part of who I was, which I had struggled with for years, had finally surfaced, to be completely dismissed by someone who (I thought) was an expert.'

Fortunately Alex was with friends, his then youth leaders, who were relatively new Christians. They were initially shocked. They'd never known any LGB people before and weren't sure what to say or do. But this uncertainty was just what Alex needed. He remembers that because they didn't know the answers 'they weren't prepared to simply trot out the usual line. Over the subsequent months and years they wrestled with the issue as I did, thinking, praying and reading up on it, and really listening to what I had to say.'

Despite this support and overwhelmingly positive recent experiences of church, his first experience of coming out has left its mark on Alex: 'I still find that I expect people in church to be negative, which is something I have to be careful doesn't stray into bitterness or negativity.' So when he returned to the same conference after a gap of more than ten years, he was initially sceptical about the extent to which this could be a good experience. But he found that attitudes had changed more than he had ever expected. 'Although those speaking fell short of condoning same-sex relationships,' he explains, 'much of the teaching appeared to point the way towards a reappraisal of the traditional line on sexuality. Exclusion based on sexual orientation was overtly criticized, and for me, the message is clear – LGBT people, their partners and their children are welcome here.'

Many churches encourage us to look to experts for answers, instead of thinking for ourselves. Both Leigh-Anne and Alex initially confided in people who they thought were experts. Both were disappointed with the outcome. Leigh-Anne *knew* she was part of the church, her own experience told her so – she didn't need her pastor to tell her she was still welcome there. Alex *knew* what he was experiencing was deeper than a passing phase, something too important to be casually brushed off.

The problem with thinking of certain authority figures as experts is that often they are not experts at all. You are the most expert about your life and your situation. You may be the one who has spent years coming out to yourself, reading, praying and reflecting about being LGB and what that means for living a life of service to God. You may be the one facing your son, daughter or friend as they nervously tell you something very intimate about themselves. The 'expert' you've approached may just, through no fault of their own, be ill-equipped to help. They may be relying on outdated ways of thinking, have an instinctive fear of difference or be genuinely struggling to give advice on a contentious issue within the church.

Finding appropriate advice can be tricky for older or more experienced Christians too. Janet and Bruce were struggling to cope with the news that their son was gay and worried about what would happen if anyone found out about his sexual orientation. Janet recalls: 'I cared desperately about what others thought, and felt people in the church would judge us.' Bruce, a church pastor at the time, asked himself: 'What would people in the church think, and what would become of my ministry?' So they confidentially approached another church leader for help. He reassured them: his church had been able to help a young man become straight and ready for marriage and he advised them against saying the word 'gay'. Janet came back from the meeting initially very encouraged, believing everything would be OK and determined never to say the word 'gay' out loud! But this advice totally denied the reality of their situation and, as Janet now recognizes, 'certainly didn't help me to move forward'. Yet, despite this, she is able to look back on this experience and say calmly, 'He is a lovely man and in many ways very wise, but I now differ from him in the area of homosexuality.'

Expert help can be really positive, but think carefully about why you are seeking it. Brenda decided to come out in church once she realized that if the love and affirmation from her church friends was dependent on her being heterosexual, then it was built on a shaky foundation and worth little. When she came out, her fears of rejection were not realized and she found overwhelming acceptance. She now believes that: 'The greatest threat to our well-being is internalized self-hatred, and an expectation that if we are open about our sexuality then people around us will respond in an offensive way, ridiculing or discriminating against us. So building up self-esteem is important in the coming out process, as then we are not so dependent on the approval of others; if that approval is withdrawn because you have identified as LGB, you will have internal resources on which to draw for a sense of well-being.' To help build up self-esteem, she recommends: 'It may be helpful to work with a suitably qualified counsellor before deciding whether to come out, someone who will give you space to explore. We have all – LGB and straight – received so many negative messages, especially from church, it would be surprising if some of us do not need to unscramble the tangle.' Simon agrees, advising: 'If necessary, go to your GP so that you can talk to somebody who is legally obliged to keep things confidential!'

Besides helping you to figure out your thinking, there are other reasons for coming out to church leaders. Michael came out to the leadership of his Methodist church to see whether they would support him to continue on the preaching rota. It was immediately apparent that they would not, but they said they were still very happy for him to help with church catering. Michael remembers: 'I felt rather second-class, and as a result I left the church.' He found his role even more restricted at the local Anglican church he then began to attend, after the curate took him aside and explained that he would not be able to include Michael in any of the public worship of the church. Our experience too is that churches will often carefully choose a line beyond which LGB people cannot become involved in church life. This can seem somewhat arbitrary: serving coffee's OK, but playing in the music group isn't; giving money is fine, but helping with church outreach is not allowed. Unsurprisingly, many LGB people also start to draw their own lines, and feel wary about offering all of their gifts to the church.

We don't want to give the impression that coming out to church leaders is always problematic. There are times when priests, ministers and leaders will be able to match their responses to your needs. Terry tells of an occasion when he managed just this. In his role as university chaplain, several students have come out to him, and one conversation particularly sticks in his mind. It was an encounter where Jesus' words about 'the truth making you free' (John 8.32) came to life for one young man: 'An undergraduate came round late one evening. He talked randomly about various things including the break-up of his last relationship with a woman. As midnight passed he began to talk again and again about "facing up to it". I kept asking gently what "it" was, but he always changed the subject. I sensed that he needed to name "it" and hear himself say the words. About 2 a.m. he finally came out to me, but was desperately afraid of telling his parents. He stood up to go and reached out for a hug. I held him for a long time in silence until he was ready to let go. About two weeks later he introduced me to his new male partner and told me, beaming, that his parents had been wonderful and loving when he'd told them.'

Coming out for good

As we said at the start, coming out in church does not usually mean making a dramatic announcement. But, at a personal and a church level, it can still have dramatic consequences, changing people's hearts, minds and attitudes towards LGB people for good.

Charles and Tom are a Christian couple in their twenties. Charles recently started attending Tom's Anglo-Catholic church where they both knew their relationship wouldn't be an issue for the leadership or the congregation. Charles explains: 'It was quite obvious from the second week who I was and they all made me feel very welcome.' They didn't have to 'come out', they simply *were* out to others in the congregation, because week in, week out, they were there in church, clearly living and worshipping together as a couple. This example had one unexpected effect: an older man in the congregation, who had known he was gay for seventeen years but never come out to anyone, came out to Tom and Charles. Why them? Because he had never before come across a gay man 'behaving like a Christian' or knowingly met a same-sex Christian couple. Meeting these two young men shifted his whole perception of what it meant to be Christian and what it meant to be LGB, bringing new hope. The encounter had a deep impact on Tom and Charles too. As Charles says, 'I've found it very powerful that just by living your life you can have a profound effect on someone else.'

Annie, whose words head this chapter, was anxious about leaving the tolerance of a big city to move to a small market town with her partner. At first her fears seemed justified when the first Bible study in their new church was on homosexuality. Gulp. But in fact, she says that this made coming out easier: 'The lay pastor told me the topic and I replied that we'd be interested in knowing the church's views as we were a gay couple. She did blink rather a lot when I said this, but made no specific comment. At the housegroup we had to obviously out ourselves quite quickly before the debate took place. People were honest but polite. As you'd expect in an evangelical church some, if pushed, would no doubt say that they feel homosexual relationships are wrong, but no one has criticized us. On the contrary, we have been quite humbled by the friendship people have shown us. We later heard from the pastor that a number of people in the church have rethought their intolerant attitudes to homosexuality because of our presence in the church.'

Jesus didn't just talk about the kingdom of God. He lived and breathed it, showed it through love and laughter, suffering and tears. That's how people knew he was the son of God. We shouldn't be surprised then if it's our lives and the way we live them that communicate the reality of being LGB and a Christian, rather than the words we do or don't say.

We believe that, in the long run, having more out and proud LGB people and their families in churches must be good for the whole church, as real people's experiences breathe life into a dry, theological argument. If more LGB people became visible role models within the church, then young LGB Christians might feel that staying in church was an option for them too. If more ministers knew that parents of LGB children were sitting in their congregations, then fewer carelessly homophobic sermons might be preached. If more LGB couples had their committed partnerships openly blessed in church, then other same-sex couples might feel able to turn to God and God's people for help if their relationships get rocky. If the insights that LGB people develop because they have had to struggle with their identity were more widely shared with the rest of the church, then straight people might benefit too from these new perspectives.

But (and there is a big but that stops this utopian vision being realized just yet) each person who comes out in church does it on his or her own. However strong you feel, sometimes staying safe is more important than challenging the status quo. Naomi is no stranger to activism, unafraid to speak out about other issues affecting her life, yet she recognizes the dilemma that many of us face when encountering prejudice: 'Had I come out when I was younger I might well have faced people trying to stop me being gay, but since then I have consciously avoided churches where that might happen. I thought for a while that maybe I should be confronting anti-LGB views, but came to the conclusion that if we all did that we'd all be exhausted. There are some people who can really do that, and other people who have other things to deal with.'

Jo came out in her thirties and also recognizes that there may be times in your life when coming out isn't an option. At college she felt that her Christian faith wasn't strong enough to stand alone and cope with rejection: 'It would have been very difficult to admit to being gay. My church was fun to be in. We had a large group of friends. I would have lost my friends and support.' Later, when she had married and started a family, the awareness of the hurt she would cause if she came out prevented her from doing so for many years.

Some people do find the strength to challenge their churches and it can be a strength born of suffering. Remember Janet and Bruce? Well, they've come a long way since that first meeting with a church leader; not only can they now say the word 'gay' out loud, but they are being prophetically provoking in their new church family: 'I have now come to a place where I want to identify with my gay Christian brothers and sisters,' says Bruce. 'I was recently asked by my vicar if I would lead a cell group. I asked him if he would be asking me to lead a cell group if I were living with "Jack" instead of Janet. He said he would not. So I said that until he could answer yes to that question I would have no part in the church's ministry team. I do try to be loving to him, but I also believe that we must take a stand when we know that abuse is going on, just as Christians did in the past when fighting against slavery.'

Coming out in church checklist

The stories in this chapter are about real experiences of coming out in church. But before you take the plunge yourself, we'd like to share with you our 'less pain, more gain' plan about how best to come out. Sally sets the tone: 'Come out in steps rather than outing yourself dramatically, and get a feel for how the church ground lies first. Confront prejudice prayerfully and with integrity, rather than with confrontational language or acts which might alienate others. Have confidence that God created you as you are and created you to be in communion with others.'

Somewhere along the line, it may be important to have a discussion with your church leader. Sometimes such a meeting can be very valuable: maybe your minister or priest has asked you to meet him or her; you're looking for advice about coming out to others in the congregation; or you want to clear the air before applying for membership or taking on a new role in the church. These next tips are gleaned from the time we have spent in ministers' offices and with vicars drinking tea in our living room, as well as from advice given by the people whose stories are told throughout this book.

- **Ensure you're both aware of the topic for discussion before the meeting,** perhaps by dropping your priest or minister a quick email in advance. This gives them an opportunity to think calmly about their response and hopefully respond with love, whether or not they agree with you. It will also help avoid the unnerving experience of being grilled about your sexual orientation in a meeting that you thought was going to be about the coffee rota.
- **Make sure your minister or priest isn't the first person you ever come out to.** The fact that homosexuality is one of the church's hottest topics may make it difficult for those in church leadership to respond in the way that you hoped they would. It's even possible that their position may be at risk if they take a particular line. So, in case you get a negative response, it's best to have at least one sympathetic friend on board already.
- **Take this sympathetic friend with you.** They don't need to say anything, they can give you support just by being there and will be able to console or congratulate you afterwards (you may need to explain at the start that this isn't your partner – unless, of course, it is). They can also help you to reflect on the meeting and to work out if you really heard what you thought you did.
- **Do your best** during the meeting to express yourself clearly and calmly – while remembering that you may get emotional and not manage to get all your words out in the right order or tone. Try not to jump to conclusions about what your minister thinks – listen to him or her too.
- **Congratulate yourself** for your bravery and head for the pub, for a coffee or for a walk with your friend. Think about whether you'd like to meet again, or whether you need to follow up with an apology or a thank you. Whether it's gone well or badly with your minister, try to get back to normal life afterwards.

But what's it like on the other side of the table? If you are reading this as a priest or minister who wants to support LGB people and their families in your care, we have some advice for you too. We're especially grateful to Sally for many of these suggestions.

- **Listen.** Find out exactly where the LGB person is in their journey and recognize it *is* a journey. People may have been hurt by previous bad experiences at other churches. These can leave them always expecting the worst and highly sensitive to comments even when no harm is meant. It also means that while welcoming words are appreciated, even these can scare people who are afraid of being let down again.
- **Involve.** See LGB people in your church as a blessing, rather than a problem. They have gifts, callings and passions to offer the church which may have nothing to do with their sexual orientation. Think about how these gifts could be given the opportunity to grow. This helps a person feel that they belong and the whole church can benefit. However, if the person feels it's right to resign membership or other church responsibilities, discuss this carefully so both of you are clear on how it is going to be handled.
- **Don't out people** unless you are 100 per cent sure that they are happy for you to talk about their sexual orientation to others in the church. If others wish to know, agree how any questions will be handled. If there are several LGB people in the church, why not see if they would like to be introduced to each other for informal support?
- **Include.** Think about how an LGB person, their friends or family will be experiencing church life – are you using exclusive language in worship or organizing activities that assume everyone is married with 2.4 children or has an opposite-sex partner?
- **Don't blame.** Don't make LGB people and their allies carry the blame for splits in the church or encourage them to be quiet for the sake of unity, especially if homophobic comments or attitudes from others are allowed to go unchallenged. Everyone deserves respect and care.
- **Resource.** Have a list of organizations that support LGB

Christians and their families ready as well as books and leaflets for LGB people, and others in the church, to read (suggestions are handily provided in the 'Where to go next' section at the back of this book).

Action

Based on your own experiences and the stories in this chapter, think about how you could make your church into a place where LGB people and their families feel safe to come out. This could be by offering a kind word to someone, proposing a resolution to become an 'affirming congregation' or 'inclusive church' (see 'Where to go next' at the back of the book for more information), coming out yourself – or even buying a copy of this book for the church library!

Prayer

Lord God, you draw us out of darkness into light, out of despair into hope, out of loneliness into community, out of fear into fulfilment. May we come out into the light of your love and know your peace. Amen.

5

Family values

Someone asked me, 'If you could change things, would you want your son to be straight?' A few years ago, my answer would have been a definite YES. However, today I can speak differently because I recognize that this is an aspect of our son that makes him who he is and I love him. Also, I count it a privilege to have had my eyes opened. Otherwise I would to this day be totally ignorant about the prejudices against gay people. (Janet)

So, you've come out to God, and haven't noticed any lightning strikes or plagues of boils. You've wrestled with the Bible and you've come out in church – or decided not to. But what about the relationships closest to home: how does a Christian family cope with the discovery that one of its members is lesbian, gay or bisexual?

In the debate about 'family values' there can be an unspoken assumption that LGB people are not part of families. That 'good Christian families' don't include LGB daughters and sons, fathers and mothers, brothers and sisters. As you know, that's not true. But this assumption can make coming out in a Christian family especially difficult, whatever the ages of the people involved. It's not helped by other preconceptions about LGB people formed by negative media stereotypes, rather than by getting to know LGB people themselves.

All families are different and in many families – Christian or non-Christian – there are already stresses and strains; broken relationships and misunderstandings exist for all sorts of reasons. When a family member comes out, it needs to be seen in that context: it may be just another pressure added to an existing difficult situation or awkward relationship. However, we would be the first to admit that coming out to our non-Christian families gave us both a much easier ride than some friends who had been brought up in the bosom of the church.

Family members of LGB people usually don't stop loving their relative once they find out about his or her sexual orientation, but they may initially be so overcome by disappointment, surprise or bewilderment that they struggle to show that love. Yet as Christians, we are called to build and maintain relationships, to forgive hurts and to find ways to continue loving each other. The stories in this chapter inspire us to believe that, however hard this may be, it is possible.

This chapter focuses particularly on relationships between LGB people and their parents (and grandparents) – from the perspective of both parents and children. On p. 88 two lesbian mothers who have come out to their children give another perspective, sharing their experiences and advice. If you're reading this as a parent of an LGB child, initial reactions of shock, worry and distress that your child has held his or her sexual orientation as a secret burden for many years may be very familiar to you. So what can parents do to show their children that they will provide a listening and understanding ear? And how can children cope when instead of love, they fear rejection?

We've divided this chapter into the most common types of parental response that we've come across, and share advice from parents and children in coping with each of these. Some parents react in all of these ways at different times, others in none of them. You never quite know what to expect, as people are complex and unpredictable. But we hope that if you recognize some of your own experiences as you read on, this advice will help you to find a new way to think about your family relationships.

Why do people decide to come out to their families?

There are many, many reasons why people decide to come out to their families, but they often boil down to two simple things: sharing happiness or ending unhappiness.

Although not yet ready to tell the rest of his family, Richard H came out to his mother and sister when he was 22. 'I'd got my first proper boyfriend, we were in a relationship together and I was really happy,' he says. When something as wonderful as falling in love happens, you want to tell the world! 'That's why I wanted to tell them, because I was really happy.'

For Christine's son, the motivation to come out was very different: a desire to end the unhappiness he experienced when keeping his sexual orientation secret. Christine explains what happened that evening, several years ago: 'Very distressed, unhappy and fearful of what the consequences might be, Adrian came out to his father and me when he was 31. The strain of "deceiving" us, he said, had become unbearable. After the tears, the hugs, the reassurances of love and affirmation, he told us that one of his reasons for not coming out earlier had been fear that, as Christian parents and because of what the church teaches about homosexuality, we might disown him.' Although this revelation was not easy for Christine to come to terms with, thankfully the fears her son had were unfounded.

'It's the end of the world'

'It isn't surprising that my parents' reaction was homophobic, as their understanding of being gay was vastly different from mine,' says IP, who can now look back calmly at a very difficult period in his family's life. The shock of discovering that their son was gay left his parents embarrassed and angry, and the stress even brought his mum out in shingles. 'They thought that I would never get a job, that I would lose all my straight friends and that I would hang out in some sort of gay ghetto. Anal sex was central to their disgust. They saw it as contrary to "natural" inclinations, a solely physical act which sounded to me very close to rape. Add to that the fact that they thought that any boyfriend I had would convince me to try group sex – basically the gay life that they thought I was heading towards was one of an eternal gang rape! It sounds ludicrous, but these elements of the overall picture – and the lack of others, notably love and affection – were obviously hugely distressing to them.'

However much parents love their children, they may be so hurt and horrified by having an LGB child that they simply can't respond in a loving way. What they hear from Christianity, or society in general, about LGB people's lives makes them fearful for their children's future. IP can see now how attitudes from inside and outside the church affected his parents' responses. 'They came from very different standpoints, and five years later, they still hold to these,' he explains. 'My mum has not changed her opinion that the Bible says it's sinful, while for my dad being gay is not sinful, but it is completely unacceptable in society.' Such beliefs can be very deeply held and as a result are very hard to shift. This was IP's experience: 'My parents turned to three members of clergy to support them in denouncing my homosexuality – all three were supportive of me coming out. So my parents ignored their views.'

Family members can be left hoping against hope that what they have heard isn't really true. IP wishes he had countered this by being clearer with his parents when he first came out: 'One of the biggest mistakes I made was to say, "I think I might be gay." By this point, I was fairly sure of my sexuality, and this ambiguity has caused huge problems further down the line. It enabled both parents to hope that I might not be gay, and also to believe that I might change my mind with persuasion.'

It seems to parents in this situation that the world has fallen apart. Some families will have to face the reality that relationships will change or end, and it will be hard ever to recover the same intimacy and trust. James N knew long before he came out that his parents would be upset to discover he was gay as same-sex relationships went against their understanding of

God's will. So he first took his boyfriend to meet his friends and his sister, rather than his parents, because he knew they would be more accepting.

Unfortunately, instead of having the time and space to tell his parents in his own way, they found out something was going on and asked his sister. Their reaction was worse than he had previously feared: 'They drove down to my university to confront me. They were hysterical – I'd never seen anything like it. My mum was crying and screaming as though in a fit, beating her fists against the table and herself. They told me I had been brainwashed by gay propaganda, that I wasn't really gay. They told me I had ruined their lives, that everyone at their church would find out and that they could never smile again because of what I had done. They said that they would have to leave church and their lives were over. They told me I couldn't come home and that they didn't want to speak to me again.

'I tried to be calm, rational and understanding while they were here. I didn't say a bad word to them,' says James now. 'But after they had left, I started absolutely bawling. It was the most heartbreaking, hurtful experience I had ever been through and I couldn't stop crying.' This is the very worst situation for a family to find itself in – but even in these circumstances, all is not lost.

'After my parents confronted me, I called my friends from back home. They drove down to my university, even though it's a long way, and came rushing in to where I lived to comfort me. In a way, it was the worst day of my life. In a way though, it was the best, knowing I had friends like these. I loved them so much for it. For me they were showing God's love, they were the ones offering hope and comfort and in doing that, they were walking in the footsteps of Jesus.'

James knew that healing would take a long time. The love and support of his friends helped him through until eventually his parents starting speaking to him again. And they do now talk regularly, although he admits that his decision to move to Australia has made their relationship a lot easier.

Christine and David's Top Tips

'A gay person might bear in mind that, for a parent, being told by their child that he or she is gay can be an overwhelming experience. Fortunately, any negative reactions are not always lasting. There should be a way to say sorry for hurtful words, often spoken in haste, and to find time and space for reconciliation,' counsels Christine.

Clearly, moving to the other side of the world is not a solution that works for everyone! While calmness and patience are not easy in this situation, they are worth putting into practice if at all possible, along with a commitment to keeping channels of communication open. Of course feelings of fear, uncertainty or pain will sometimes be long-lasting, but the most important thing is to maintain relationship in spite of these feelings.

Parents may need reassurance that their child has not suddenly changed into a person they don't know. For David, the breakthrough was meeting his son's same-sex partner. He advises other parents: 'Give yourself a chance to get to know your child's partner; you might actually like them. In our case, we did; that eased things a lot.'

'What did I do wrong?'

Most parents don't believe it's the end of the world when their child comes out, but many still find that their instinctive response is to blame themselves, either for having an LGB child or because their child hasn't felt able to confide in them before. This is completely normal: parents never grow out of feeling responsible for their children, or worrying about their well-being.

While Bruce is now totally accepting of his son being gay, his first reaction was paralysing guilt, based on myths and preconceptions about LGB people: 'My understanding at the time was that homosexuality was a perversion brought about by wrong family relationships. That is, a remote, uncaring father figure and an oppressive dominant mother figure. Although this didn't really match our profile, I knew that there had been too many times when I had been off looking after the church where I was pastor and leaving the bringing up of the children to my wife.'

And while Bruce worried that he might have failed as a father, his wife Janet began to doubt her ability as a mother. 'My first reaction was to run and tell our son I loved him,' she says, 'but also to ask him where we'd gone wrong – what awful sin had we committed, and to try to work out how to get things fixed. I was distressed to realize that my son knew from around age 11 that he was different, had hoped it was a phase he was going through and later had prayed he'd be delivered from it. He had been going through something on his own for years and thought he might never be able to tell anyone. I'd hoped I was a good mother and yet I had been totally ignorant of all of this.'

Alex's Top Tip

'It's nobody's fault you're gay. Some people in the church still cling on to outdated ideas about same-sex attraction being a symptom of a poor relationship with your parents, often your dad. It isn't. Make sure you let your parents know that when you come out to them – that'll save them a whole load of guilt as well. I think we often massively underestimate how much time and space we owe our parents to come to terms with their child's sexuality, and just how much of an effect it will have on them.'

Churches sometimes pass on myths and misconceptions about LGB people as if they are God-given truths. Parents who blame themselves for their children's sexual orientation may need to hear from church leaders, from friends – and from their children themselves – that it is not related to anything they have done and that being LGB is not a matter for blame at all. The World Health Organization, the Royal College of Psychiatrists, the American Psychiatric Association, the American Psychological Association, and all legitimate scientific evidence agree: being LGB is a fact of life, not a disease, disorder or death sentence.

'So what's the big deal?'

Like many of us it took Alex some time to accept being gay. When he came out to his parents at 19, he believed that same-sex relationships were wrong and that celibacy was his only option for the future, and he told them so. He knew they would be supportive and compassionate, despite coming from a conservative evangelical background, but was still surprised by their level of acceptance. 'In actual fact, they were rather more progressive than I was,' he says now, 'although they were upset I had kept it to myself for so many years, and deprived them of the opportunity to support me through it.'

Far from being ready to condemn their LGB child, some parents can be more relaxed about their child's sexual orientation than even their child is, especially if they have already encountered LGB people or issues in a different context. 'My dad's first reaction was to suggest putting me in contact with a gay vicar he knew,' recalls Alex. 'And my mum said she didn't think that celibacy was necessarily a very good idea. When I protested that the Bible was very clear on this, my dad suggested that maybe the point of being Protestant was the freedom to look at the Bible afresh.' Their support continued as Alex's own views shifted over time. 'Years later, when the time came for my partner to be introduced to my parents, it was clear from day one he was part of the family, and it's been that way ever since.'

For some parents, once they have accepted the news themselves, the desire to support and stand alongside their children goes beyond a personal level. It motivates them to march at Pride, campaign against prejudice and powerfully show the church and other Christians through their words and actions that families with LGB people are equal members of the body of Christ.

Christine and Paul D's Top Tips

'Among family and friends, my son has found love and acceptance as a gay person in ways that he never thought possible, or would have known, if he had not had the courage and the strength to face the risks involved and leave the closet,' says Christine. Parents who see their child struggling or unhappy, but are unsure why, are often keenly waiting to be given the opportunity to offer love and support. While it takes courage to come out, the acceptance of parents and other family members can really help the person coming out to accept themselves.

Paul D adds: 'I urge all parents with LGB sons or daughters to affirm their children constantly, and to make that affirmation public. It's fine to say that you are still on a journey with the implications of your grown-up child's sexuality. I assure you, your child is on a similar journey. If you have a Christian faith and struggle with the tension of your child's sexuality and what you have been told the Bible says, then find out for yourself. The internet will give you some fresh approaches and help you to find some resolution.'

'I'm worried because I love you'

Many parents worry that being LGB is going to be tough and will mark their child out as different, even if it is totally accepted within the family. They accept and love their child and want to protect them from the prejudice they see 'out there': 'I had always wondered if Rachel was gay, so when she told me she was, I was not surprised but pleased that she felt able to share it with me,' says Vivien. 'It's not an issue within our close family unit and we are all supportive – now it's the total norm for us. My main concern was, and still is to a certain extent, that not everyone is accepting, and my worry is for the hurt and problems that some people's attitudes could bring.'

While the stories elsewhere in this chapter show just how dramatic coming out can be, it wasn't the case in Paul D's family either. 'Our son Chris joined my wife and me in our garden where we were relaxing on a sunny afternoon. He told us that he was gay and had been aware of this reality for a long time and wanted us to know,' explains Paul. 'The odd thing was that it was an unemotional time – we both took the view that nothing had actually changed – we still loved both our sons, that wasn't going to change. I suppose if I were honest, I would have preferred the situation to be different, but only because his road would inevitably be a harder one than if he were not gay.'

Peter H's Top Tip

Peter's mum was determined to understand and get over her preconceptions about gay people. 'She said the most profound thing that she learnt was that gay people are normal, or as normal as everyone else,' he tells us. If homophobia is something parents imagine when their child comes out, then they will naturally be worried. Of course homophobia does exist, but LGB people are better equipped to survive it if they have unconditional support from their families. The parent who worries about their child is likely to have already given their child the internal resources to cope with prejudice.

'I knew all along!'

Some parents know all along that their child is LGB, perhaps even before their son or daughter is able to articulate this for themselves. Maybe you are one of them, reading this book to help you prepare for the conversation when it comes.

Before Gwilym came out, his mother had her own ideas about what might be going on. He explains what happened: 'In a conversation she started about my "interest in gay culture", my mother mentioned that she "had never met such a bunch of queens in all her life" as when she met my father's friends from college where he and they had trained as Anglican priests in the late sixties.' Now, having met some of them, and agreeing with his mother's assessment, he still wonders, 'I am not sure if she was setting them up as positive role models or as some kind of warning from history of what I could end up as. Maybe one day I will ask her.'

For Bruce, the awareness that his son was gay came as a huge shock at first. 'It never even occurred to me in my wildest dreams that we could ever have a gay son,' he says. 'We were good Christians weren't we? We brought our five children up to strictly follow the scriptures. It didn't happen to people like us. But one day, I felt God show me that our middle son was gay and that it was OK. I went into a spiritual tailspin. At the time I didn't tell anyone – feeling it was confidential information.'

Bruce now recognizes how helpful it was to have been able to overcome most of his negative emotions in private before his son told him he was gay. He then felt able to reach out to his son and decided to speak to him on a day when he seemed troubled in himself. 'I said, "I think I know what you are going through and would be happy to talk it over with you." He didn't respond at the time but did come out to me some months later. By God's grace, I was able to hug him, tell him I loved him and that everything was going to be fine.'

It can be a great relief, for both parents and children, that the time of waiting and wondering is over. Parents who always suspected have had time, perhaps over several years, to come to terms with any difficulties *before* their child comes out and are now ready and able to give their full support.

Lily's Top Tip

'To someone just finding out that their child is LGB I would say "don't panic". Think before you act, say or do anything – and by and large don't act, say or do anything differently from how you would have before. If your child comes out to you, thank them for trusting you with the information. If you find out some other way, keep the information to yourself for a while. If you feel the need to talk to someone about it, make sure it is in a confidential situation – it is your child's decision as to where, when and to whom they come out and you should not pre-empt that decision.'

As if it never happened

When Rob came out to his parents, shortly before leaving home, it was in his words 'very, very dramatic'. His mum cried and cried and his dad refused to believe him, claiming that he would be straight in six months.

And what has happened to all this emotion, months later? 'We never really talk about it now,' says Rob. 'It's the big elephant in the room. I don't need to bring it up because I don't really have any gay friends, and I don't have a partner, haven't had any for a long time, so it doesn't come into things, it's faded away.'

However, Bill's experience shows that silence, and even hostility, can develop with time into understanding and restored relationships. 'When my partner and I first lived together my mother was glad I was living with a nice young man,' says Bill. 'When we bought a house together, she visited and saw our double bed. After that I had a lot of insinuations about when I was due to get married, when I was going to have children and how I should visit without my partner.' At this point, Bill realized that this situation could not continue. His mother's denial of this important relationship left him feeling emotionally vulnerable. At last he found the courage to visit her on his own and says, 'My mother and I had an indirect conversation, obviously painful for her, in which we came to an understanding.'

Since then, actions have shown themselves to be more important than words. 'When my father died, my partner was very supportive and my mother, who had been very close to my father indeed, appreciated that,' explains Bill. 'Usually when we visited, my partner was given a double bed and I was notionally assigned my old bedroom, and would creep in to him at night. When we visited during my father's last stay in hospital we shared the same room and my mother took it for granted as other family members needed the other rooms. We have always shared a bed there since.' And when, in his fifties, Bill and his partner entered into a civil partnership, his mother was right there beside them, a vocal supporter of their commitment. He says: 'My mother is registered blind, so we were not sure whether to ask her to sign as my witness. But when we asked her at the end of the ceremony, she almost leapt across the room in her eagerness to do so, and signed with great difficulty because of her sight.'

James W's Top Tip

A family not acknowledging that it includes an LGB member can be hurtful. It can feel like a denial of that person's identity or a door closed in the face of further discussion. James knows that his family are not going to start publicly or privately acknowledging his sexual orientation any time soon, but has found a way forward through accepting his family for who they are. He says: 'I have accepted their inability to discuss the issue and they have accepted me as I am and have shown me an overwhelming sense of support and love. It just goes to show that actions speak louder than words.'

'Fine by me, but what shall we tell your grandma?'

'Will we ever tell great-grandma?' wonders Bruce. 'Probably it would be kindest not to, but on the other hand – she's a great fan of Dale Winton! Until our culture changes and gays are fully accepted in our schools, churches and society in general, the coming out process will never stop.'

'Most people in our extended family now know,' adds Alex. 'But one debate still rages on – should we tell the grandparents? They're 92, farming folk, and conservative with both a small and a big "C". At the moment we're all fairly convinced it would be better to not say anything – they have met my partner on several occasions and know we share a flat, but just think we're jolly good chums. Arguably that's a closer approximation to the reality of our situation than if we were to tell them we were in a gay relationship, which for them would mean "they're going to hell", "they're living in sin" and "they're going to get AIDS". Or are we depriving them of a chance to share in a really important part of our lives?'

Once parents and children have broken the silence, whether it went well or badly, a hurdle's been crossed. But the tricky decision of whether or not to come out to others in the family still remains. Deciding how to come out to wider family members takes time and thought. Parents and children have to feel comfortable with who is being told what and how. Even when you think you know what the response is going to be, there can still be surprises.

Peter H's mum dried her tears and joined a group for families of LGB people, finding it helpful simply to realize that she was not alone. And it's had quite an impact! 'Now she's going through a stage of outing me to everyone,' says Peter. 'It feels a bit unnecessary sometimes, but she's like, your uncle and cousins know now . . . ' But it was left to Peter himself to tell his grandma. 'I expected my grandma not to take it so well because she's more religious. But she immediately said, "well, it doesn't make a difference to me" and told me about how her experience of working with the Samaritans had made her realize that you can't judge people. It made me realize that you just can't tell what people's reactions are going to be.'

Bruce talks about the stages that many parents have to go through before feeling comfortable about telling wider family and friends. 'Coming out is an ongoing process for parents as well,' he explains. 'Once your gay son or daughter has come out to you, your times of coming out are just beginning. Of course, you stay firmly in your own closet until you have gone through the various denial/self-blame/grieving stages and are, finally, free to honestly appraise where you stand on the issue.

'So, first of all you come out to yourself . . . "Yes, I am the proud parent of a gay son/lesbian daughter." This was more difficult for us because of our strict religious background. Then, with your child's permission, you can be free to come out to close friends and family members. But what then? Not everyone has a right to know. It isn't always necessary or even appropriate is it? Well no, but then unexpectedly, a well-meaning friend shouts across to you in the pub, "Has your Johnny got himself a nice girlfriend yet?" And it goes suddenly quiet. "No, but he has got a really nice boyfriend," you reply. The silence deepens for a while as the penny drops and slowly people resume their conversations.

'You do this when you are ready, not before. Some parents may never get there. For most of us a time comes when we feel free to be ourselves and tell it like it really is. If that loses us some friends, then they were best lost.'

Vivien's Top Tip

'When telling people about your son's or daughter's relationship be positive. Say "I am delighted to let you know . . ." This leaves less room for a critical response and I find people respond positively. But if they don't, then don't get into arguments. Accept people's comments and prejudices even if they hurt.'

Spotlight on . . . coming out to children

Sally was single when she came out to her 12-year-old daughter, but had decided it was time to start looking for a relationship. The principles that she found useful could help any LGB parent – and their children – whatever their situation.

1. Don't force the issue; let the conversation arise naturally, in a relaxed situation. In our case my daughter made some

---

smart comment and it gave me an opening for the discussion which I took.

2. Respect the fact that your child may want you to be subtle, particularly in front of his or her friends. My daughter was concerned that if her friends knew then she might get bullied. I talked this through with her and reassured her.

3. Think about what you have around the house when your children have friends coming round. On one occasion I had a mailing from an LGBT organization on my desk and my daughter commented she had friends coming round and asked me to sort my desk out.

4. Realize that some of the issues your child raises might have nothing at all to do with you coming out. They could be because of general parenting issues (like 'mum's thinking of dating again') which could apply whether you were gay or straight.

5. Give them time to get used to the idea as a natural part of life without making an issue out of it. By just leaving it as 'that's the way it is', but answering her questions honestly, my daughter was able to get used to it.

Jennifer's son was 16 when she came out to him. She describes it as one of the hardest confessions she's ever had to make, but doesn't regret it. 'When I told him, he looked at me and said: "You're my mother and I love you." We now joke about the type of woman I'm attracted to. He doesn't particularly think much about my taste. Once I told my son and other family members that I was a lesbian, they were very supportive and acted no differently from when they thought I was straight.' She adds, 'I strongly believe I have the right to be me and celebrate difference and uniqueness in a world that is full of so much prejudice.'

The parenting of God

> 'As a mother comforts her child, so will I comfort you.'
>
> **Isaiah 66.13**
>
> 'It was I who taught Ephraim to walk, taking them by the arms.'
>
> **Hosea 11.3**
>
> 'For you created my inmost being, you knit me together in my mother's womb.'
>
> **Psalm 139.13**

There are many powerful images throughout the Bible and Christian tradition of God's loving parenthood. There are promises to comfort us as a mother comforts her child, to guide us like a father teaching his son or daughter to walk and there is reassurance that we are known and loved by God from our first moments of life. A relationship with God gives us a strong foundation to start seemingly overwhelming conversations, survive apparently impossible challenges, and work towards healing the most painful hurts. As parents and children whose relationships may be changing, we thank God that we can hold onto these promises when we are distressed and in need of comfort, or confused and in need of guidance.

Action

Have a look through some family photos – the ones in your wallet, on your phone or in an album. Are there family members with whom you still have issues to resolve, whom you want to thank for their support or whom it's simply time to catch up with? Now's the time to pick up the phone, send an email or arrange a visit.

Prayer

God our comforter, creator, parent and guide, you knit us into families and your image shines out through those close to us. May your love living in us help us to listen patiently, support generously and love wholeheartedly. Amen.

Special features

We have tried to pack as much as possible into the nine chapters of *Living It Out*. However, four issues stood out as being distinct and demanded greater attention than we could give them within the main chapters. The following special features allow four of our contributors to share their experiences in greater depth and explore crucial issues facing many LGB Christians and their allies: mental health, being LGB at school or in a church youth group – both as a student and as a teacher – and engaging with the media.

A JOURNEY THROUGH DEPRESSION

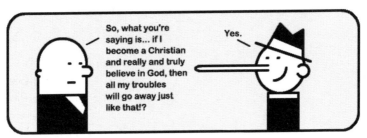

The Revd Pinocchio

Kate first came out as a teenager and shortly after became a Christian. Now at university, she tells her story as someone who has 'journeyed through depression holding Jesus' hand'.

I became a Christian six years ago at the age of 16, during my GCSE exams and in the middle of a very difficult time in my personal life. I had begun coming out to people over a year earlier, to a mixed response from my friends, and I had just been diagnosed with depression, having attempted to kill myself. Bringing Jesus into this mix was going to be the best thing I ever did, and at the same time one of my greatest challenges.

Before I became a Christian I had been attending a youth group at my local Church of England church for three months. On the night I finally chose to commit to Christ, I had told myself that I was seeking something that didn't exist, and had decided to leave the group. As it happened, I had to be there early and ended up sitting in on the service. I couldn't tell you who was preaching, or what they preached about, but I left the church that night knowing that I had accepted Jesus, and that I was at the start of a long journey. I was elated.

Intellectually, I knew life wasn't always going to be easy, but a part of me did believe that it was going to be easier from now on. At the same time, I found myself in a position where I could no longer dismiss what had been said to me by Christians about my sexuality. I immersed myself in the Christian debate about sexuality; asking questions of my Christian friends and reading everything I could lay my hands on about the Bible and homosexuality. Walking with Christ was already proving to be more complicated, and more conflicted, than I had foreseen.

As time went by, I decided to seek guidance from members of the youth leadership team at my church. I was fortunate enough to be in a church with a very supportive and faithful group of leaders; and I received a great deal of support from them. However, the message was clear: if I wasn't healed of my homosexual inclinations I would have to remain celibate in order to honour God. I felt very strongly at the time that this was not right for me, but I continued to pray and to struggle. In the three years from becoming a Christian to leaving for university, this was how I dealt with my sexuality on a day-to-day basis.

It is perhaps not surprising that I continued to struggle with depression. My GP prescribed various antidepressants but, although they alleviated the daily symptoms, the problem didn't go away. I was seeing a psychotherapist once every two weeks, but often felt worse when I left her office. By the time I was 17 I had been self-harming through cutting myself for two years, and I was developing severe bulimia. It is to the credit of the leaders dealing with me, and to a very good friend who helped me to confide in them, that I didn't go entirely to pieces during this time and that I kept my eyes on God as much as I could.

By and large, the next couple of years continued on the same course. I continued struggling, but began to feel more and more isolated. People at church assumed that my depression was due to my continued struggle with my sexuality. I was still exploring the debate within Christianity about the status of LGBT people in the church – and, more importantly, in the eyes of God – and I was beginning to believe that whatever I decided to do about relationships, there was nothing to be gained by being 'cured of homosexuality'. I was miserable at church, and saw no way out of the void of depression. I blamed the church, but didn't want to leave.

After a bit of church-hopping in my first few months of university – and having walked out of a service when a well-known preacher gave thanks to God for those who were standing up against homosexuality – I began to attend meetings of Young LGBT Christians. By this time, I had joined the university's LGBT society and was determined not to let my sexuality prevent me from finding a church. Eventually someone mentioned the Metropolitan Community Churches. I was uncomfortable with the idea of a church founded in the LGBT community, and worried I would find myself in a place where God came second. I could not have been more wrong, and I also found out what it was like to be fully accepted into a community as who I was, depression, scars, irritating habits and all. God called me there as part of the healing process, I do believe that, and without them I don't know if I'd have got to where I am today.

I am just about to complete my BA in archaeology, classics and classical art, and despite struggling off and on throughout my course with depression I am hoping to graduate on schedule. I am no longer having regular treatment, and am entirely over both my eating disorder and my long-running self-harm problem. Of course things aren't all perfect, and I still find that I have bad days, but I pray the worst is behind me.

My story is unique, and not a model that can be applied to all young people with depression, but I would like to give one piece of advice to those who find themselves having to help people cope with mental health problems. Please try to remember that depression is not a sign that someone is not right with God, it is an illness that needs careful treatment. If someone feels accepted by their community as a whole person, illness and all, it might not cure them but it will make the whole process much more bearable for all.

COMING OUT IN THE CLASSROOM

Reuben, a 16-year-old, tells his story of coming out to friends at his Church of England school and church youth group.

At age 14, year 10, I started to come out to my friends; on a Monday, I think it was, I told five of my closest friends, plus a few whom I simply felt empowered to tell, that I was gay (and that's not changing any time soon)! Now, I'm sure everyone who reads this book will know that kind of news spreads like butter in a mechanized sandwich factory – very fast indeed. So of course by Tuesday my entire year group knew, by Wednesday the whole school knew, by Thursday the staff knew (or at least that would explain the sudden appearance of Stonewall and Young LGBT Christian posters in classrooms and corridors) and by Friday, I suspect the blooming bishop knew! Initially, I was bothered by this; I didn't want everyone knowing. It was for my close friends' knowledge only – but I very quickly came to feel that honesty was an awful lot easier; besides anything else, it meant I didn't have to hold my tongue so often, for example when a meltingly beautiful guy walked past, or when the discussion turned to homosexuality in Religious Education lessons or at Christian Union meetings.

I realize that at my school I'm lucky – when I told the chaplain about my first boyfriend, she was almost as excited and pleased as I was. Although Section 28* has in the past prevented the issue being faced ('Thatcher, Thatcher, freedom snatcher!'), there is now hope that I will be able to be an LGBT 'peer listener' to whom any student can come to discuss any issues they have around these matters. My request to do so has led the school to seek training for the existing peer listeners. So I am in a much better position than many of my peers: my school is wonderful at handling these issues, but, as in any faith school, there are individuals who hold hateful views. I have been subject to arrogant, 'holier-than-thou', presumptuous recommendations of celibacy from staff, and both 'But how can you be gay AND a Christian?' and 'Well, I believe the WHOLE Bible' from ill-educated, overly evangelical students.

But this attitude of theirs is powerless – wrong and vastly unjust, yes, but powerless – because I know, we know, that God loves us. Why does he love us? Because he does. Just . . . because! I am not saying I don't get angry with them – I DO; but they cannot get between me and my God. I know that it's easier said than done, but I try (and usually fail!) to just praise God and blank it.

Youth groups? Well, they vary. It tends to depend on the youth leader. If you can gauge how likely they are to bite your face off, usually that attitude will be consistent among the

---

* Section 28 of the Local Government Act 1988 stopped local authorities from 'intentionally promoting homosexuality' or 'promoting the teaching in any maintained school of the acceptability of homosexuality as a pretended family relationship'. Although no prosecutions were ever brought, some teachers were afraid of discussing LGB issues with students for fear of losing state funding. Section 28 was repealed in Scotland in 2000 and the rest of the UK in 2003. (Information taken from http://en.wikipedia.org)

young people. How out can you be? Usually it is a case of if you can't be totally out in your youth group, you'd be best staying totally closeted. Church youth groups will probably always be tricky. My advice would be just be careful, really! Listen to God, let him guide you.

If you're a leader in a youth group at a church and someone comes out to you, BE SENSITIVE!!!!!!!!!!! These people are baring their souls to you – it's about a lot more than sex! If you're going to discuss it collectively, the number one rule is to do your research and find out the details of the misinterpretations of those infamous verses; number two, to make it abundantly clear that a loving relationship between two people of the same gender is NOT a sin, and, number three, to be as relaxed and comfortable as possible around the issue – it should be almost a non-issue!

WORKING WITH YOUNG PEOPLE

Anthony shares his experiences as a gay man who has been both a teacher in a faith school and a youth leader in his local church. Now in his thirties, he is training to be an Anglican priest.

As a teacher, I never made a secret of being gay. Students are naturally curious about their teachers and often ask questions that can be personal. I was fortunate during my training years to have a sensible head of department who gave me the following advice for teaching sex and relationship education: 'Answer all questions except those about your personal sex life, sex with animals and fetishes, especially if they are the same.'

This I extended to all questions. I have never regarded being gay as being about my 'personal sex life', although, invariably, this was the next question my students asked, and I came to accept the fact and respond, politely, that what I do or do not do is none of their business. I found that it was the next set of questions that were the most interesting.

The majority of the students who attend the Catholic comprehensive school where I taught have a reasonable understanding of the church's teaching on most issues. They, therefore, are aware that being Christian conflicts, somewhat, with being gay, and from this arises discussion about truth, humanity, love, justice – in fact, those things that Jesus talked about during his ministry. I like to think that being so open has given students in the school a good example of a gay person and not a stereotype. I am encouraged by those that have the courage to come out at school and by their general acceptance by their peers.

Among the Catholic staff, parents and priests there is a ground-level compassion for people and their lives that contrasts with the doctrine from the Vatican; they live with the two in tension, persistently remembering and recalling that we are called to live lives centred on Christ's sacrificial love.

There have, of course, been times of sorrow among this joy: this life we live is a bunch of roses with the thorns intact. Yet the pain has never been due to the faith we live, rather to the homophobia and heterosexism cultivated in disaffected young people by their parents at an early age. I want to make it clear that these young people who strove to cause me pain and distress were themselves suffering, as so often is the case with bullies. They were invariably at the bottom of the year group and bottom of their peer group. It is our challenge, as Christians, to hold those who would cause us the most pain closest in our prayers. It is important that school procedures are followed should they cross a boundary, for they are trying to bully: if one attempts to be 'nice', they will take further advantage. One should, in love, treat them the same as every other student would be treated when he or she tries to bully a teacher.

I have also worked in a secular school, but I preferred working in a faith school for I found greater support for myself as a person and as a Christian. Being out at school was my choice. I know and understand that this is not for everyone and I continually affirmed to students who asked me about other gay teachers that it is their choice to tell them, not mine. I have found the most important factor in being a good teacher is being yourself to your students and loving them for who they are regardless.

Being gay is part of who I am, part of me. Being gay, therefore, affects my spirituality, my physicality, my personality. Christians are not dualists who separate the spirit (good) from the physical (bad), but recognize that God has given us everything and it is good. I can deny my 'gaiety' as much as I can deny my right knee or my love of trying to understand the world through science. I am, therefore, out with some of the youth groups I work with.

I said 'some', not 'all', and this is important. Unlike at school where all the young people who ask these questions are teenagers and are trying to understand their own sexualities in light of others, the young people I work with at church fall within a larger age range. Discussions around sexuality rarely arise with children under 11, and, when they do, it is best to field these back to the parents. Since I make no secret of being gay, the young people at church accept it when they discover it from their peers in the youth groups; the great advantage with these groups is that they cross age groups and year groups, and young people in year 8 talk to young people in year 11 more than they would at school. The questions that arise are similar to those at school, but have less of an 'edge' since they are talking in a different relationship than teacher/student. Needless to say, discussions must remain within appropriate boundaries and with child protection in mind. I can, however, go into greater depth with the young people at church about biblical interpretation and how being gay has affected my relationship with God.

Working with young people is and hopefully always will be a joy and a privilege. They are alive and imaginative, longing to learn and soak up all the world has to offer and challenge it in all it does. They are persistent in this challenge, but for those of us who can meet this head on (and I think everyone can with the right frame of mind) working with them is its own reward.

ENGAGING WITH THE MEDIA

Brenda has spoken out about LGB Christian issues through the press, local radio and on TV. Here she shares her experiences.

My first involvement with the media was not exactly of my choosing: my name had been given to a BBC reporter without my consent. I was in fear and trembling during that interview, expecting to be asked questions that I couldn't answer; I phoned a friend for advice on the topic and memorized a couple of key points. That seemed to do the trick, I survived the experience and now use every opportunity to broadcast a positive LGB Christian message.

I have found local radio stations, BBC and independent, welcome a newsworthy story, and are by and large sympathetic in interviewing. Not all presenters are Jeremy Paxman or John Humphrys! They usually create the space for the interviewee to say what they want to. You have to decide in advance which one or two points you want to make, and keep coming back to them; you don't have to answer every question posed if it does not lead you back to your chosen points. Just keep talking.

If you are involved in an LGB Christian event of any kind, my advice would be to promote it through the media. Write a short press release, no more than one side of A4 double spaced, in simple non-jargon language with a catchy headline and a quote from yourself or a key figure in the event showing why it is newsworthy. Add contact details at the bottom and email it off to local radio stations and newspapers a week in advance; then follow it up with a phone call. If you are invited to give an interview and make a reasonable job of it, you may well find that you are contacted in future for comment on a relevant news story.

You may want to comment on a news story relating to LGB issues, in which case letters to the church press, or a call to a radio phone-in may give you a platform. Contact details for press and radio can be found on their websites. Always be brief, don't assume your readers and listeners know anything about the subject, and always be polite, however provoked you may feel. Where possible give the 'good news' positive angle, rather than just arguing against a negative story; take the lead.

Usually radio presenters have been reasonably well briefed on the topic, so can ask sensible questions. But this is not always the case. I was once in a discussion about civil partnerships with a local conservative clergyman, when the presenter suddenly blurted out 'Well, how do you know God exists anyway?' We were both stunned into momentary silence; not that easy to marshal the arguments for the existence of God in thirty seconds at seven in the morning. At least we had found some common ground, even if not with the presenter.

6

No longer the only one

The first time I worshipped with other gay or lesbian Christians was so liberating for me, I really felt God in that place, in that community of people where I belonged. Finally those two pieces of my life that never seemed to fit together, started fitting. (James N)

Looking back now, I'm not sure why I was so frightened when, as a teenager, I (Sarah) clipped a short article about an LGB Christian group out of the newspaper and tucked it in the back of my diary. I'd look at it every now and again and think about getting in touch. But it was at least three years before I did. Was it the fear of somebody else knowing I was a lesbian that made me wait so long? Or the thought that these Christians who thought being LGB was OK couldn't *really* be Christians? Or the worry that once I knew other LGB Christians I would have to start fitting a stereotype and stop being me?

I know I'm not the only one who's felt this fear. So how and why do people overcome it and search out LGB-related groups – Christian or otherwise? We've found that it's often a strong desire to belong and to find people who understand, that pushes people to confront their fears. It can be just the same for families and friends of LGB people who want to make contact with others in a similar situation to themselves. Finding this safe space is particularly important if you have lost a previous place of safety through being rejected by family or church. But we know that meeting and getting along with new people can be difficult, confusing and downright scary, so we hope that this chapter will assist in smoothing your way.

Each section heading is a tried and tested tip or piece of

advice that may be helpful when finding and joining a group, illustrated by quotes and stories from the personal experience of our contributors.

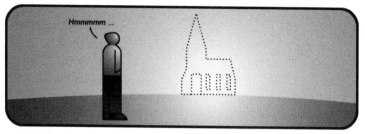

A building is no longer a place where I find church.

Feel the fear – and do it anyway

If you are having difficulty accepting your sexual orientation or that of a family member, simply walking alongside others who are travelling the same path can help bring healing, but it can be a difficult or frightening step to take. Janet was struggling and still in denial about her son being gay when her husband suggested attending a group for families and friends of LGB people. It was a long time before she felt ready to go along, but she needed to take that time. Now she describes their decision to go as 'one of the best we've made'. Finding a group of people who understood and accepted them enabled Janet to express painful and pent-up emotions: 'The first time I went along I think it would have been OK if I'd just cried the whole time, because there's been no expectation that I have to act in a certain way but just be myself. That in itself is a very healing thing.' Her husband Bruce also pays tribute to the group's 'many caring people who have wisdom that has been born out of pain'.

Christine took her time after her son came out before joining a similar group and found friendship and encouragement when she did so. She knew she had many questions, and initially began to resolve these through long conversations

within the family, between herself, her son and her husband.
'For some time, just talking together was all that I needed,'
she explains, 'but as the months passed, I began to want to
meet other parents who were in a similar situation and to meet
more gay people – Christian and non-Christian.' The care and
understanding that she found in that support group inspired
her to continue attending its meetings in order to help other
members. She also lends a confidential listening ear on its tele-
phone helpline.

Shop around

Many different groups exist for LGB Christians, their friends
and allies, so shop around. A list of groups that our contributors have found helpful is included on p. 160. Many joined lots
of different groups before finding the place where they feel at
home. Others continue to remain involved in different places
in different ways. The campaigning agenda of some groups in
reforming and challenging the church as a whole can be an
inspiration to some and a real turn-off for others, who prefer
a more pastoral approach. So you might need to shop around
and try out several groups before you find the one that's right
for you.

For some of you, the most important thing might be finding
people with a shared denominational background or theological stance, for instance Roman Catholic, Quaker or evangelical. After all, being LGB doesn't necessarily mean having
to redefine everything about your faith, so the place you feel
comfortable and accepted may be with those with whom you
share a common background. For others, the opposite may be
true. Peter C was brought up in an Anglican/Methodist tradition, but discovered a new richness through joining an ecumenical group of young, LGBT Christians, where he encountered
incredible diversity. 'Through the people in that group,' he
says, 'I have learnt about retreats and festivals, Unitarians,
charismatic evangelical worship, convent life and transsexual

priests . . . In many ways, therefore, this group has helped me to be a more well-rounded Christian.'

Meeting, in person, people living LGB and Christian lives also helped Peter feel more secure about being gay: 'I sensed that the people I met were just as successful as the straight congregation in leading Christian lives. What is more, the couples that I met showed me that God is not only willing to work, but *enabled* to work, through LGB relationships. And for me that led to the conclusion that if God does work through relationships held together partly by LGB desire, then those desires that I had been suppressing could be God-given and used to further God's purposes.' For him and many others, the name, the denomination, the purpose or even the age range of a group don't matter, it's the people. Finding friends, role models or a partner can be a strong motivation for joining a group.

Be willing to give and to receive

Joining a group also gives people the opportunity to support others by using and developing their gifts. Margaret used to be very involved in her local congregation. She was the sort of person who keeps the church afloat. After her children came out, she decided that she couldn't stay within the church, but still wanted to serve God. By joining several groups devoted to struggling for justice for LGBT people both in and outside the church, she could contribute to helping change the church and continue using her gifts. This includes using her professional counselling skills to supervise a helpline service for LGBT Christians, their friends and families.

Once he was outed at his local church, Jim was no longer encouraged to use his gifts in that setting but, through LGB friends he made after starting university, he unexpectedly found an opportunity both to develop his own confidence and to use his gifts – even ones he didn't know he had. 'I got involved with the LGB society,' he explains, adding wryly, 'In the first year I got more involved than I intended – I was elected officer towards the end of that year. When the election results were announced, I thought "12 months ago I didn't have the confidence to tell a stranger I was gay, now here I am, I've got to start preparing for when the new freshers arrive!"'

Be realistic

At their best, groups can be familiar and diverse, pastoral and political, a place to give and to receive, meeting different needs at different times. They can become a source of companionship and friendship, church in the widest possible sense: a community in which to worship, to love and serve God together.

However, as you'd expect, no group is perfect. Just because you've got one thing in common, doesn't mean you'll all necessarily get on. So it's important to keep a healthy dose of realism. Gwilym, who's been part of several groups, tells it like it is: 'They are mostly the same mix of oddballs as the rest of the church. I have had the privilege of knowing some wonderful people, but have also had to deal with the same amount of politics, infighting and difficult people as in every other bit of the church. Gay Christians are not a superior race; wisdom, revelation, and insight about the future of the church has been given to some of them – but in no greater measure than to straight Christians.'

People often find such groups when they are hurting or vulnerable, so it takes extra care and commitment to build a place where all feel safe and welcomed. How aware, we wonder, are those of us within such groups of how people outside perceive us? Do the strong friendships that we value so much make us seem like an exclusive clique to others? Do the shared language and experiences of the group make newcomers despair of ever fitting in? Each of us is faced with the challenge: how can we make the groups that we're part of into truly welcoming places for all?

This is not easy. What we say and what others hear can sometimes be two different things. Elaine talks about how at a

Christian festival, where the LGB community has a strong and friendly presence, she was struck by the openness and welcome that she received from the people who identified with this community. Yet she felt there was an air, particularly among the young men, of an eagerness to please that hinted at an underlying fear of not being found acceptable. She says: 'I remember during one late-night conversation when I said that I'd have to be going – there was a disconcerted moment, when I realized that the two men I was speaking to were not sure whether to take this as rejection, rather than tiredness.'

While there are advantages in creating a separate safe space for LGB people, their friends or families, to explore issues unique to them, many feel strongly that if any section of the church is cut off from the wider family of Christian believers then everyone loses out. Anthony, who talks about his experience as a teacher and youth leader in a special feature on p. 97, set up and ran a specifically LGB youth group once. He wouldn't do this again because he believes that 'this is segregating ourselves, and the young people of today do not need it. Young people need the safety to explore themselves and the world that our youth groups in our churches provide. We should, as a family, talk honestly. And our young people are part of our family and should be included in the discussions, for they will surprise us and inspire us.'

Be open-minded

This talk of different groups is all very well, but if you're reading this in a tiny town with one LGB night a month in a seedy club, what kind of choice can you really make? Relying on what you can find locally can lead to some unexpected, but potentially positive, experiences. So we advise looking widely and being open-minded about what you try. The first group that I (Rachel) went to was one for LGB Roman Catholics which had advertised locally. For a Baptist like myself the prospect of attending Mass (should I or shouldn't I take communion?)

and following a liturgy that everyone knew (and I didn't) was daunting, even without the need for secrecy. But in the end it didn't matter. These people were warm and welcoming and not nearly as fazed as I was by the denominational difference.

Go online

The internet has radically changed the way in which people find information and meet each other, making geography a much less important issue. And the kind of fear that I (Sarah) experienced when first looking to meet other LGB Christians is reduced if you don't have to meet people face to face straight-away, or ever. Instead, you can get to know them online and ask all those embarrassing questions you'd otherwise be too shy to ask. Surely, it's worth a go.

For Peter H, especially while he was still living with his parents, the internet meant he could find help and support not just nationally but internationally. He says 'one of the things that I found most helpful in the early days of questioning my sexuality was an American group with an internet chat room. There I was able to say to people "how do I even know that I'm gay, how do I know for definite?" It was helpful to have those conversations over the internet, to realize that there were people who had gone through something similar to what I was going through. Although it's really confusing and hard to deal with, I knew people had been through it. That was really encourag-ing.' Other contributors have recommended YouTube, where seeing real people talking about their experiences and their beliefs is potentially more powerful than reading text.

Peter's experience encouraged him to find ways of promot-ing such groups to the people who most need them: 'I know a lot of gay Christians who go through this experience of feeling like they're the only one. Once you realize that organizations like this exist, you really want to be able to promote them. It's so hard to do because, in certain churches, there's no way you can get that message to people. Or you might be able to say it once, but you'll never be let in again, so pick the right morning!'

Now, most of us will already be pretty savvy when it comes to the internet, resisting the daily email offers of cheap Rolex watches, Viagra and mail-order diplomas. But Simon has a few less obvious pieces of surfing advice to help with your online search for groups: 'Bear in mind that some browsers may store terms that you have searched for,' he warns. 'It can be an issue if other people use your computer or are in the room when you type in "G" and "Gay Christian" comes up.' Simon also recommends using an anonymous username on any forums: 'This is particularly wise if, like me, a few not-very-personal details can narrow you down to very few people, for example if you live in a small town or village or have an unusual occupation.' And finally, he advises taking care how you choose your search terms and being discerning about what you may find – 'Be ready to come across ANYTHING!!!'

Resist the pressure to be someone you're not

There is another kind of group that LGB Christians encounter: ex-gay ministries and the organizations that promise a 'cure for homosexuality'. While you may find some genuinely caring people there, such groups can not only be deeply damaging, but also spectacularly unsuccessful. Robert was encouraged by his vicar to attend an ex-gay weekend. He remembers it as 'very frustrating. On one hand I had to try to conform to the weekend – to change from being gay to their norm – while on the other having feelings towards the other attendees. When I returned, to my church's shock and horror, I still had the same desire for men.' After what his church saw as his 'failure', Robert felt increasingly marginalized and finally changed churches. At his next church, he felt God calling him to something new: to set up an LGB-affirming group in the parish. 'I wrestled with this idea for a few months, and at the end of the day God won,' he explains. This group ran for three years.

Its successor, Haven, is still running and celebrates its fifth birthday this year. Within the ex-gay movement Robert felt pressurized to be someone he wasn't, but he says that many experience Haven as 'a place just to be yourself'.

Some, like Alex, turn to the ex-gay movement because it appears to be a simple answer to a complex problem. 'When I was about 14, I saw an Oprah programme on TV where some people claimed they had once been gay, but following an ex-gay residential programme, were now happily married with kids,' he says. Encouraged, he went into his local Christian bookshop the next day, and surreptitiously sidled up to the 'Christian Living' section in search of a book that would explain how he too could be 'healed'. A book on coming out of homosexuality seemed to fit the bill, so Alex threw caution to the wind and bought it.

'Fortunately for me (in retrospect), it didn't make much sense even then. It told the story of two ex-gay people, a man and a woman. The woman had been a very butch lesbian, wearing dungarees and no make-up. Redemption came in the form of a woman named Candy at her church, who took her under her wing and showed her how to put on make-up and wear more feminine clothes. This was clearly positioned as a key part of her leaving behind her "gay identity", and yet surely being a straight woman was not about knowing how to use mascara? Slightly disappointed, I moved on to the man's story. His major breakthrough was learning how to read the sports' pages so that he could confidently make conversation with other men at church. That put the tin lid on my interest in the ex-gay movement. My dad, a robustly masculine, well-adjusted and happily married man, was not interested in the sports pages. I could kind of imagine myself managing to hold down a successful marriage with a woman, once I'd sorted out the gay thing, but I knew I was never ever going to be remotely interested in the sports pages either.' Alex now lives with his male partner of five years. The ex-gay book still sits on their bookshelf as a reminder of what might have been – and it is rare to find either of them reading the sports pages.

Unlike Alex's 24-hour flirtation with the ex-gay movement, Jeremy knows it inside out. He devoted his life to running an ex-gay organization, until he realized that this approach wasn't working. He started to find that the people who left the programme generally found 'a solid basis of love, faithfulness and commitment' in same-sex relationships, but those who remained committed to denying their sexual orientation were left with 'a deep sense of personal failure coupled with profound disappointment in God'. Jeremy made the brave and powerful step of turning his organization around so that it became an affirming place where people can be 'really gay and really Christian'.

However, despite the damage he now feels that ex-gay organizations can do, a feeling echoed by many of the contributors to this book, Jeremy recognizes that they can help some people to articulate their sexual orientation for the first time and break through their isolation. Richard P first met other LGB Christians through Jeremy's organization. He was motivated to join by 'a desire to learn from those who had been through such a struggle', thinking that it was 'surely a waste to repeat the futile efforts of the past'. In that group, and others he has joined since, Richard found 'a network of gay Christian people through which I have been freed to explore faith. While religion once caused me to be consumed by worries about my sexuality, my sexuality has freed me to explore faith more deeply.'

The bringing together of these two aspects of life – a Christian faith and an LGB sexual orientation – alongside other people is perhaps one of the most valuable experiences that can come from being part of a group. This wholeness is something you are unlikely to find elsewhere and may even have found being actively discouraged. Charles describes the feeling of completely belonging somewhere for the first time: 'I had always felt different, the odd one out. Having met Christians at university who would not accept me because of my sexuality, and LGBT people who could not understand how I could be a Christian and gay, joining an LGB Christian group was a huge revelation. The love and support that the group members show each other is a true depiction of God's love, manifested to us through the love of friends.' When people worship together, openly, with an awareness of each other's struggles and joys, it can be an incredibly emotional experience, one that allows people who have been hiding from God to start to be honest again. While not everyone will enjoy being part of a group, we all need friends who understand us. Building an informal network of support through existing friendships and people you meet along your journey can be just as necessary and just as enriching as joining an organized group.

Find the strength to go out

Rather than being a place to hide from the world, a good group builds the strength, confidence and self-esteem of its members so that they can come out and speak out. When I (Sarah) overcame my initial fear and went to meet other LGB Christians, I sat in petrified silence at the first meeting before quickly bolting for the door. But I pushed myself to try again and now I know that some of the best friends I've made, and the most rewarding things I've done, have come as a direct result of plucking up the courage to go to that first meeting. The two of us wouldn't have met, let alone thought of writing this book, unless we had been able to talk and meet with other LGB Christians. That's part of our story.

Everyone has their own story of how the love, support and example of others has helped in their personal journey. Many of these are told within this book. Peter H says that his mum was only confident enough to tell the rest of the family that she had a gay son once she started attending a group for friends and families of LGB people. Sarah I found the courage to speak in her church about her experience as a lesbian because she knew there were many others in the denomination who felt the same way as she did. Bruce benefited from the understanding of other parents of LGB children and now feels equipped to help and encourage other parents who are going through trauma. We're sure that you have your story too.

Action

Visit the website of one of the groups listed in the 'Where to go next' section at the back of the book. On this occasion, instead of finding out how the group might be able to support you, think of a way in which you could support it, perhaps through a donation, signing up to a newsletter or in prayer.

Prayer

Emmanuel, God with us, you came to share our life. We pray that you would join us as we join together, sharing our laughter and tears, arguments and struggles, secrets and celebrations. Amen.

7

Career path Christianity

During my time as a minister, living alongside lesbians, gay men and bisexual people, hearing their stories and supporting their cry for justice, led to me being thought of as a friend by some, an enemy by others, and an infernal nuisance by many. Yet it continues to be life-enhancing and gospel-affirming. (John)

This is the big one. The controversy that has rocked the church. Jeffrey John and Gene Robinson are the names that everyone knows, yet behind the media headlines are countless LGB men and women balancing on a knife-edge to fulfil their calling to minister.

There's no lack of LGB people in or considering ordained ministry or full-time Christian work, although few denominations officially ordain 'practising' LGB people. However, many potential contributors with compelling stories to tell and wise advice to give were scared of being identified as this would put their jobs at risk, or they were already under too much stress to have the energy to contribute, making this a very difficult chapter to write. So we're grateful to those who have been bold enough to share their stories and reflections to help those LGB clergy, their partners, families and supportive straight colleagues who wrestle daily with living a lie or witnessing to an uncomfortable truth. Many clergy face this dilemma. Should they be true to what they believe is right – even if this entails lying or hiding the truth from church authorities? Or is it better to accept and live by teachings that they don't agree with? Or are there other, maybe more creative, ways forward?

But a sense of vocation is about much, much more than a call to ordained ministry. As Christians, we are *all* called to build God's kingdom, whether in business, in education, in the voluntary sector, in bringing up children – in fact, wherever we find ourselves. Although the stories in this chapter show there are particular challenges facing ordained ministers, there are LGB Christians in all kinds of other jobs. This chapter looks at how we can all negotiate the intersection between work, sexual orientation and faith, and live out our calling.

Where is God calling you?

LGB people who feel called to work for the church may end up having to find other ways of ministering than as a parish priest or church pastor. Working for Christian organizations is a popular choice as an alternative to ordination because it means that your private life does not have to become public and you are protected by law from discrimination. There is no issue around whether your partner comes to church with you or lives in the vicarage as a never-quite-defined 'friend'. There's no 'don't ask, don't tell' chat with the bishop and no fear of being found out by your congregation.

We've both been employed by Christian organizations or local church projects at one time or another and have been surprised how few people have had an issue with our relationship. In fact, the most awkward situation we encountered was when a member of the congregation at the church where Rachel worked hadn't quite understood the nature of our relationship and assumed that Sarah was her daughter! We hasten to add that there are only four years between our ages. When we organized a week of 24-7 Prayer for a group of local churches, even churches that were unwilling to have a lesbian couple as part of their worshipping community were happy to take part in the project. Although this is not the case with every church or Christian organization, it does seem that LGB laypeople can often avoid the controversy and discomfort experienced by their ordained brothers and sisters.

Oscar has wrestled with such issues throughout his career, and God has led him to different conclusions at different times. He initially left a career in advertising, in which being gay was not a problem, but being a Christian was 'the love that dare not speak its name', to become a member of a religious order complete with vows of poverty, chastity and obedience. What a contrast! He presented himself to the Jesuits as a candidate who was gay and at ease with his sexual orientation, but also prepared to be celibate. The response was more positive than he had expected. 'The questioning I received was not about my sexuality,' he says, 'but rather about how easily I could change to a celibate lifestyle, especially after having been in a committed relationship. The questions seemed to be the same as they would have been had I been straight and coming out of a committed relationship with a woman.'

The British Jesuits' attitude of acceptance, while not shared by all the Roman Catholic Church, meant that Oscar did not have to lie and was accepted by his gay and straight Jesuit brothers for all the gifts he brought, including his sexuality. He explains: 'I could be Jesuit and celibate and gay and all those identities would coexist. And my prayer life as a Jesuit, especially through the regular silent retreats, confirmed that this was where God wanted me to be.'

However, after six years he chose not to pursue ordination as a Jesuit priest. Three experiences in particular shaped his decision and gave him new perspectives on the challenges faced by gay men wishing to serve in ordained ministry within the Roman Catholic Church.

The first was the experience of denial, during the time that he was sent to live and work in a refugee camp in Uganda. Although a grace-filled experience where Oscar learnt much about God's love and the joy of serving others, he was told frequently that there were no homosexuals in Africa. 'So not only could I not claim an identity as a gay Roman Catholic,' he says, 'by this definition, no one could claim one. I survived, and thrived, but the experience taught me that the "universal church" does not have a universal attitude of love towards those whom God has made gay.'

The second was of rejection. A Vatican document, signed by Pope Benedict XVI, strengthened the hand of bishops who felt that gay men could not be priests by instructing them to question potential ordinands and to reject those with 'a deep-seated homosexual tendency'.

The third experience was more personal: 'I realized that I could not live a life of celibacy. This is not because I don't believe that celibacy is a good thing and that for some men and women it is a gift from God that helps them in their ministry. But it is a gift, not an obligation or a burden. Some priests can live it happily and humanly. I realized that I could not – not because I was gay (I know many gay celibate priests) but because I am what I am. I am now discovering how it is that God wishes me to live my life, gay and Roman Catholic and no longer celibate, but nonetheless called to build God's kingdom.' Oscar's journey continues, he now works for a Catholic charity, where he is comfortably out as a gay man.

Some, like Peter C, have found that their LGB sexual orientation has changed the way in which they decide to carry out their vocation. What may have begun as a feeling of limitation, has become liberating. He describes the blessings of a sexual orientation which for him entails not having children: 'I feel no pressure to be in a position of relative financial and physical security in ten years' time in order to raise a family. I am therefore able to work in an unpredictable profession and in unpredictable areas. While parents rightly have to concentrate their care on their children, God has put me, along with other childless individuals, in a position to minister more fully with other people in society, showing the nurturing love of a parent in a different way.'

For many Christians working outside a church environment (that is, most of us), talking about personal faith is more likely to cause a change of subject or embarrassed silence than any sexual revelation. Alex has found that in the companies where he's worked, he's never encountered so much as a raised eyebrow when people realize his partner's male. This is more than can be said for being a Christian at work: 'Once people have got to know me well enough to realize I'm not about to force them along to an evangelistic coffee morning, they tend quite simply to be baffled,' he says. 'Why would anyone be a Christian in this day and age? How can that make sense and what on earth do you get out of it? In my workplace, being a Christian is seen as an eccentric and possibly morally suspect life choice. Being gay is just who you are.'

Following a call to ordination

A few years ago we had a shocking realization. Virtually all the LGB Christians we knew were either leaving the church – or exploring ordination within it. So why this explosion of potential LGB ministers and priests, seeking to serve a church which is at best ambivalent and at worst hostile towards them? Daniel and Anthony have both responded to this calling, and, as gay ordinands within the Church of England, are able to share with us their decisions and experiences.

Anthony chose to reject secrecy and deception early on his path to ordination. 'My priestly ministry began as an idea over a decade ago and has sat deep in my gut like a rock in a pond, sometimes covered and hidden, but revealing its weight from time to time,' he says. 'I've taken my time over accepting this call, but at no point did I make a secret of my sexuality.'

Why did Anthony wait so long? Partly because of the difficulty of 'accepting authority and being obedient, accepting that even should I have a relationship, it cannot be a sexual one'. He is clear that his obedience is a deliberate choice, not a calling to celibacy or an agreement that celibacy should be a requirement for LGB clergy. It does not affect his commitment to continue to pray and work for change and acceptance.

Daniel made a different decision. He started by trying to be totally transparent, but was soon faced with a difficult choice:

'I was out at church and enjoyed the support of my vicar,' he explains, 'but my diocesan director of ordinands made it clear I could not progress any further unless I broke up with my boyfriend. I was not prepared to do this, so my vocation was put on hold.' His strong and confirmed sense of calling and his knowledge that the Church of England document *Issues in Human Sexuality* forbade same-sex relationships for clergy naturally put great pressure on his relationship with his boyfriend.

One day, while still struggling with the tension he felt between his calling and the official position of the Church of England, he heard a comment that made him see things in a whole new way, that 'the calling of God is one; that God's calling on one's life is not in tension, but a unified whole'. He describes this as the time when 'the penny dropped that God is not calling me to be a priest in spite of my sexuality, rather God is calling me to be a priest with my sexuality. The whole of my life is raw material through which God's grace manifests itself.' He realized that he no longer felt that the tension existed within himself, but that it existed within *Issues in Human Sexuality*.

This realization meant, for him, that 'I must appear to abide by *Issues in Human Sexuality* in order to be selected and ordained as an Anglican priest. I must present a facade for official purposes, while hiding my private life. This kind of subterfuge is detestable to me, and I find it disgusting that the Church of England should create a situation that demands duplicity and hypocrisy from its clergy.'

Both Anthony and Daniel's decisions involve some element of compromise, trying to make a stand while recognizing that the church, and the world, are not perfect. They are both decisions that require careful thought and prayer, and have a personal cost. They are not made lightly.

Most denominations take the line that an ordained minister is not permitted to be in a same-sex relationship, but this becomes much more complicated when it comes to bisexual ministers. Bedford outlines the following scenario: 'A bisexual man gets ordained to the priesthood. He has a wife to whom he has been married for a number of years, and there is no way he would be unfaithful to her, with either a man or a woman – he is, in effect, living as a heterosexual. However, he still openly identifies as bisexual, and prior to settling down with his wife he had sexual experiences with men – none of which he regrets. Should this priest be allowed his pulpit?' We've never heard this kind of issue acknowledged in discussions before, let alone resolved.

It's not just those entering ordained ministry who face difficult decisions. Partners and other family members may not have heard the call, but they too face challenges. Chris experienced this when his boyfriend at the time started exploring a calling to go into the Anglican priesthood. His partner was very clear that it was perfectly fine to be gay and a vicar, and that their relationship wouldn't be affected in any way. However, Chris knew that the big metropolitan evangelical churches where his partner wanted to minister were generally not keen on people being openly gay, never mind them entering the priesthood.

This put pressure on the relationship and on Chris's own ability to be involved in the church. 'Our relationship was always kept quiet, and in the end it was just easier for me to leave our church because we were spending the whole time worrying about people finding out we were a couple,' he says.

Growing up gay in a vicarage family gave Gwilym a particular relationship to the local church which any 'child of the manse' will recognize. He describes 'a tendency towards a quasi-public role – the "office" of vicar's son – which gives rise to the cultivation of a public and a private identity even before any ideas of sexual orientation are taken into account'. As the vicar's son, he was conscious of not wanting to become an issue within his father's ministry, explaining that, 'I always tended to leave out sexuality in the construction of the public identity. This public church life meant that the family has been the major context of genuinely wholehearted expressions of faith identity. The whole of my extended family is a church family and it has been a broadly affirmative space – one of my sister's godparents is an openly gay priest, and more recently my aunt had Jeffrey John preach at her first Mass after having been ordained.'

He urges LGB people facing the decision about whether or not to go forward for ordination to think carefully about what the implications would be, as well as the risks associated with being outed. 'How are you going to manage the separation of your working life in the church and your gay life? What about the potential for paranoia to grow about people working it out?' he asks. 'Will this lead to you asking gay friends or your partner to be straight when they visit you, or will you just not let them visit? And having taken this all into account, ask yourself: in working for the church you should be giving of yourself, and is that really possible if you are not being honest about who you are?'

Being honest about who you are is more than just being comfortable with your sexual orientation, as Gwilym found when he was considering whether or not to continue in full-time Christian work himself. He explains: 'The aspects of the work I enjoy most, and am best at, are being taken forward by evangelical churches, which would have meant working in a context that was different from my own tradition (the Catholic end of the Church of England). I think I could have done it – except they would have been places where my sexuality would have been ignored or actively rejected. This was a double bind. I could have coped with being an evangelical for a few years, but a straight evangelical would have been too much!'

Truth and grace breaking through

When Sarah B was selected for ordination in the Anglican Church she was single and full of insecurities about her sexual orientation. But by her second year of training, she felt able to acknowledge her identity as 'a lesbian and a beloved child of God' and to tell her friends and fellow students. Despite having chosen to attend a liberal college where she thought being LGB would not be an issue, she found that 'the college did not celebrate my coming out as much as I thought it would. I quickly learned the lesson that you could be gay and in the church, but there were certain rules you needed to follow. The most important rule is not to be publicly out.'

After her sexual orientation came under scrutiny during her first years of ministry, following this unwritten rule became impossible. She spoke to a diocesan official about her long-distance relationship with a curate in the USA, and was then told that she had to come out to her bishop. 'In one way I was so relieved,' she remembers. 'I would no longer have to use coded language and to feel that I was splitting myself in two. But coming out put extra pressure on me. Very personal questions were asked, and constant enquiries about my "life-style" were made. The level of questioning made me feel like my relationship was unclean and inappropriate. Prior to my ordination to the priesthood, the bishop gave me a list of conditions I had to meet in order for him to ordain me and for me to remain in post. These included not living with my partner, being "celibate", and not publicly disclosing our intentions to have a civil partnership. I had been told I could have a "lodger" if I was discreet, but we were not prepared to go down that route.'

Now coming to the end of her curacy, she feels that she cannot again accept a position which will ask her to hide her relationship. 'When my current post ends in a few months, I will move to the USA to live with my partner and take a position as a trainee hospital chaplain,' she says. 'My partner is currently serving a curacy in a parish where she can be out and where our relationship is supported. We are open to the possibility of one day returning to England, but right now it is hard to imagine coming back to serve in a church that has hurt us so much. Even if it means that we struggle to find parish work, we need to be true to ourselves and the communities we are serving. How can we preach the message of God's unconditional love when we are not living it out? We have to minister with integrity if we are going to minister at all.'

Honesty is also a crucial issue for Paul T. He's spent five decades as a Roman Catholic priest, giving of himself in his parish, in prison and hospital chaplaincy and in social justice work, yet he has never come out to church authorities despite being with his male partner for over 30 years. How has this self-giving been possible? 'The one very important way in which my sexuality has contributed to my ministry has been that having to hide my true self from people, which I have felt to be dishonest, I have compensated for this by an almost obsessional desire to be honest in every other way. I have tried resolutely never to toe the party line, but always to say what I truly believe. For instance, I have never hidden my disagreement with the official attitude of our church on contraception or the remarriage of divorcees. I have tried to be honest on dogmatic issues, giving my opinion, but saying that each must decide for themselves.'

Feeling that he had to compromise his honesty in order to serve as a priest made Paul acutely aware of the value of honesty and openness. He describes that experience as 'a valuable gift' which has contributed enormously to his ministry and his relationships with people. It's Daniel's realization lived out again: the whole of life, sexuality, struggle and all, is the raw material through which God's grace is manifested. Even the negatives, difficulties, compromises and rejections. Even those. Nothing is wasted.

The same was true for Jim. Brought up in the Salvation Army, he was active in the youth network and played his flugel in the band. It was where he felt he belonged and as a teenager he started to think about becoming an officer. That plan changed when he was outed and, in such a close-knit community, the news spread fast. No longer allowed to play in the band, or even wear the uniform, being an officer was now certainly out of the question. At the time he was devastated: 'I was planning on being an officer. I hadn't made any thoughts on what I wanted to do jobwise apart from that. Of course that all fell through, my world collapsed, and at the time I thought, "where am I going to go? What am I going to do?"'

But, looking back, he too sees that grace at work: 'Now I can see the positive impact: I've had a wider experience of life. If I was to go into officership now, if it ever became possible, I would have a better understanding of life in general, not just the narrow closed-minded view I had at the time I was outed. It's changed the direction of my entire life, not just my faith, because I've had to go through that challenge and find my own ground in the church.'

Even negative experiences bring with them new understanding and insight, as well as strengthening the commitment to stand up for deeply held beliefs in the face of opposition.

Straight ministers taking a stand

While it is clear how prejudice or fear of prejudice affects LGB people in ordained ministry and their families, the impact on their straight colleagues can be less obvious. But the following story from Terry shows they too can find themselves in difficult positions, once they start to ally themselves with LGB issues and concerns.

'During the 1990s I always wore a red ribbon on my stole when leading worship. I knew so many people who had recently received an HIV diagnosis that I wanted to feel close to them during worship. I remember one World AIDS Day visiting a new church for Sunday worship. I strode out to the front and turned to face the congregation. By the time the first hymn ended there was silence and everyone was staring at me in a less than friendly manner. As I began the words of welcome several people got up and walked out. Several more people didn't receive communion from me. Afterwards one man who'd walked out met me at the church door. He asked why I was wearing 'that filthy thing' and what I meant by desecrating his church. I tried to explain but he refused to listen. As I left the church that morning I began to realize what my gay

124

friends and colleagues could be up against if they contemplated coming out in a Christian context and how far the church had to grow before it could learn to offer authentic ministry among those living with HIV/AIDS.'

Lily, who describes herself as 'a good vicar's wife', knows how hard it can be for LGB people to come out to those in church leadership. 'Sometimes in the past friends have not felt able to trust us with the truth and so have gone on denying their sexuality in our presence,' she reflects regretfully. 'It saddened us that they could not be honest and it damaged our relationship with them, but we always tried to keep the door open and keep in contact. With hindsight perhaps we should have tried to put them in touch with someone who could help – but this was difficult in an establishment such as the church where a word in the wrong ear could damage someone's standing and prospects.'

John, whose quote heads this chapter, retired in 2006 after 41 years as a Methodist minister. He served as a circuit minister, a university chaplain, as Connexional Secretary for Continuing Development in Ministry and as the first Team Leader of the Formation in Ministry Office. For readers who aren't Methodists, this means he was a big cheese in the Methodist world. He has also championed acceptance and inclusion of LGB people within the Methodist Church at every level, and continues to do so even in retirement. This has included proposing a resolution which 'recognized, affirmed and celebrated the participation and ministry of lesbians and gay men in the church' and called on Methodist people to 'begin a pilgrimage of faith to combat repression and discrimination, to work for justice and human rights and to give dignity and worth to people whatever their sexuality'. He was hugely gratified when this resolution was passed resoundingly by representatives of the Methodist Church at their 1993 annual conference.

It was a single intimate conversation with a fellow minister that started John on this path. 'One extraordinary encounter affected me deeply,' he recalls. 'It was the day a gay minister talked honestly to me about the agony and ecstasy of his sexuality. At the time, I found this encounter profoundly disturbing. I had to face up to my own fear and aversion to those whose sexuality is different from my own. Yet this was to be but the first of many such encounters; they were gifts of grace.'

If only we could all be more open to these gifts of grace and to celebrating our encounters with difference. To recognize that the Bible's story of leadership, from Deborah to David to Peter, is filled with the unlikeliest of individuals who, however strange it seems, are nonetheless God's intended choices. Yet it is hard to see the bigger picture when LGB ministers and those exploring the call to ministry get caught up in lies and half-truths, in fear and secrecy. However, away from the headlines and the limelight, these ministers are getting on with their jobs: administering church life, taking services and comforting and challenging their congregations.

Taking into account all the difficulties they are likely to face, should LGB people continue offering themselves to serve the church in ordained ministry? It's not an easy decision to make. But there is one thing we have no choice over: however we express it and whatever job we do, God is calling each of us to a life of love and service. We don't have to wait until we're totally sure where we're going, but to step forward in faith today and see where God leads us.

Action

Being an ordained minister can be a tough and lonely job at times. Think about those you know personally in this situation and think of a way in which you can offer them practical support this week.

Prayer

Jesus, good shepherd, you tell us that one day all secrets will be revealed and all things will be made known. For clergy, those considering ordination, those working full-time in lay ministry, and those who love them, may this promise be a source of hope and bring an end to fear. Amen.

8

Love and marriage

I increasingly longed for a close relationship with another man. I wanted a proper relationship and not just physical intimacy. I couldn't see what was wrong with that. Why could love be wrong just because it was between two guys? (Simon)

I find it strange that marriage is talked of as the Christian and biblical ideal. The Old Testament ideal would appear to be polygamy, and the New Testament ideal would appear to be celibacy. (Bill)

The two of us met in 2001, started going out in 2002, moved in together in 2003, married in 2005 and our daughter was born in 2008. None of this sounds particularly radical, yet in our teens and early twenties neither of us could have imagined our lives taking such a conventional path. As this chapter goes on to show, many churches find that accepting and affirming LGB people who are in or looking for committed relationships is a very radical step.

Do you agree with countless love songs that suggest life is incomplete without a romantic, sexual relationship? Do we simply want girl-meets-girl (or boy-meets-boy) romantic comedies which are otherwise identical to the boy-meets-girl ones? Or can we question our culture in the light of our faith and offer alternative models of relationship? After all, as Bill points out above, biblical and Christian tradition don't offer a resounding endorsement of marriage, having much more to say about living in community than living in partnership. The stories about friendship in this book show that non-romantic relationships are also incredibly important. So why a separate chapter on 'love and marriage'? We chose to include this chapter because partnerships are a source of joy and nourishment to many people, and same-sex couples have long been denied recognition of their love. The lack of external support and role models make it difficult for LGB people to embark on relationships confidently and leaves friends and family confused about what same-sex relationships are really like. Perhaps 'gay marriage' is such a controversial and threatening issue within the church because so few people actually know same-sex couples. Help is needed.

In any bookshop you'll find shelves of self-help and etiquette titles – both secular and Christian – on love and relationships, with topics ranging from finding a partner to planning a wedding. But they don't cover everything. What if you're LGB, newly out and wondering about dating and your faith? Or if you've been asked to your first same-sex wedding and are not sure how to respond? We suspect you won't find a book to help. That is, until now. The following chapter is packed with advice and personal experiences from people who can answer these very questions.

Meeting and dating

What?

There is a long tradition of celibacy within Christianity from the New Testament onwards, particularly for priests or members of religious orders. Celibacy is often seen as a calling that enables a person to free themselves from family commitments and dedicate themselves to serving God. Some churches still encourage LGB people to strive for celibacy because they see all same-sex relationships as sinful, but other people, including ourselves and many of the people who share their stories in these pages, feel differently. We believe that while celibacy is a valid calling and a choice open to both LGB and straight people, so is partnership. Therefore the church should be supporting LGB and straight people who feel called to celibacy in the same way, instead of pressuring straight people to find a marriage partner and LGB people to remain permanently single.

Chris decided fairly soon after coming out that he wasn't going to be celibate. 'The decision of whether or not to be celibate is a very important choice to make,' he explains, 'but I wasn't in a position to make that choice because I didn't know what I was choosing against – I didn't know what it was like to be in a relationship. So I decided to give dating a go.' But he cautions that nurturing other relationships is vital too. 'If I were to give any advice to people coming out, I'd say to concentrate on developing friendships rather than romantic relationships. When you first come out you will be very lucky to make a relationship work for a period of time because your entire life is in such a state of flux. But the friendships I made in that first couple of years of coming out have helped me grow as a person and settle into this new life I have carved out for myself. By all means date and see what happens and figure out what is important to you in a relationship, but never neglect your friends.'

Time for a reality check. Whether you're straight or LGB, much of what you expect from your first relationship is the same. You're just waiting to be swept off your feet by Prince or Princess Charming and live happily ever after, right? But while straight people often have their first relationships in their teens, so hit reality pretty early, for LGB people that first relationship is likely to come later, in their twenties, thirties . . . or even as late as their eighties! So by that time expectations may be even more unrealistic.

Richard P brings us back to earth: 'Churches seem to think we're engaged in all manner of exotic activities, as part of the rumoured "homosexual lifestyle". It seems we're all having sex at every opportunity. By this standard, many of us gay people are leading rather quiet, boring lives! We really do just the same things as anyone else – work and come home, go to the supermarket, do the ironing, cook dinner, watch TV – and would like to do all this with someone special. This isn't nearly as exciting as the lives I hear that we lead.'

There is more to a relationship than sharing everyday activities. Karl explains how falling in love enriched his faith: 'It was when I first experienced being in love and being loved that I was convinced that God loved me as I was, not as I should be. This made me more confident in my trust of God.' Not bad to find out that a same-sex relationship can bring you closer to God – especially if you've previously thought it can only bring misery and a slow descent to hell.

Who?

The next question in your mind may be whether to look specifically for a Christian date. This was certainly the advice given by the church youth groups that we both grew up in. But as they also told us that mixed-sex dating was the only option, can we trust them on the Christians-only thing?

Having decided to 'give dating a go', Chris found that a relationship between two Christians could be overwhelming. 'Whether to only go out with Christians is a really difficult question,' he says. 'There are the advantages of having a shared faith and being able to talk openly about God things. But coupled with this is the fact that gay Christians generally have a lot of issues around how they have been treated by the church or by their Christian families. So you may end up just talking about problems all the time.'

Karl found positive benefits in having a non-Christian partner, helping him to explore and question his own attitude to life: 'My partner is agnostic but has a contemplative attitude to life – it interests me more to partner someone with different beliefs than the same beliefs.'

However, having a difference in beliefs can sometimes mean holding different priorities and making different life choices. Gwilym cautions that, although a relationship between a Christian and non-Christian can work out, it can bring its own difficulties: 'As a person of faith you will at times be irrational, will allow yourself to suffer without justification, will continue to maintain relationships with those who oppose you, will give without thought of reward, will invite odd people into your life – the list can go on and on. These are increasingly rejected by "secular" society. Your partner may struggle with these "abnormal" behaviours if they are unable to place them in the context of faith, and when they get to the end of their tether and say "it's me or the weird people from your church" you will find yourself in an impossible position, because deep down you will know that the weird people will win out in the end because that's where Jesus is.'

We know that churches can be exceedingly unhelpful when it comes to same-sex relationships, the only guidance offered being 'don't'. So Alex was lucky in finding one of the few evangelical churches in London which was very accepting of LGB people. In a fairly ropey relationship and wondering whether same-sex relationships were ever really a good thing, he went to his vicar for advice: 'He suggested I break off the relationship. This I was expecting, but then he suggested I look for someone better, maybe even a man who shared my faith. This I wasn't expecting.' But that left Alex with a new question to worry about: where to look.

Where?

Simon admits it can be tricky to meet your dream date or potential partner: 'The only way I have found to meet a lot of other gay people is via specific gay groups and events. However, these can be fairly scarce, especially in a small town, and don't give you much time to get to know people properly. I'm concerned I'll seem like I'm hitting on people, when all that I really want is to get to know someone enough to see if I may want to ask them out.' All the same, we do know people who have made close friends and even met a life partner in this way.

There are some churches, often the more Anglo-Catholic ones, where you will find significant numbers of gay men.

Although this is one way to meet people, Bedford, a bisexual man in his twenties, has found this not to be without its hazards: 'At a church function an older gentleman decided to make my acquaintance, and we engaged in the sort of conversation where one person takes a step towards the other, who then takes a step backwards and, to make matters worse, by the time I had reversed the entire length of the buffet table he decided to broach the subject of women in the ministry. "You're not in favour, I trust?" he asked me. "Well actually," I replied, "I'm in favour of women in general. Some of my favourite girlfriends have been women." At that point he not only decided to curtail the conversation but left me alone for the rest of the evening, leaving me free to chat up several young men who'd already made their escape from him.'

Thank God for the internet, which can bring together people who may otherwise never meet (a Christian lesbian between the ages of 25 and 30 in your neighbourhood . . . unlikely. On the internet . . . why, there are thousands!). You may meet the perfect person, but it's likely you'll face disappointment along the way. So, of course, you need to take care and keep your expectations realistic when looking for love online (visit www.getsafeonline.org for more tips on internet safety). Michael used the internet to make contact with possible dates but took things slowly: 'I met a young Scotsman on one of the less scary gay social networking sites, and the two of us drew together during many, many phone conversations over the course of nearly four months. I had established early on that he was a Christian, but that wasn't of prime importance. It was more important that he had the right attitude of love and patience.'

Now, we're not getting any commission on ticket sales, but we met at Greenbelt Christian Arts Festival, as did . . . well, pretty much all the same-sex Christian couples we know. Alex and his partner are one. Following his vicar's advice to look for a Christian partner, he thought that the Greenbelt seminar 'Can you be gay and Christian?' could be just the place to look. Five years later, he's planning his civil partnership with David, who had gone to the seminar with a similar thought in mind!

'My faith is a huge part of my life,' Alex says. 'While I would never have ruled out a relationship with someone who didn't share that faith, it has been wonderful to be able to be part of the same church family, to be able to talk to one another about God, and to pray together at times.'

How far?

So, you've found your date. Now it's time to address another church youth group debate: how far can you go? In general, there is a lack of guidance for Christians trying to conduct sexual relationships in keeping with their faith and with the realities of contemporary life. This is not just an issue for LGB people.

Annie remembers that her church youth group was very pre-occupied with physical expressions of affection and with the perennial How Far Can We Go debate. She says: 'We watched teaching videos on sexuality for teenagers that advised lustful teens "Don't Touch What You Haven't Got". It would be unfair to blame these for my same-sex youth group experiences, but it's safe to say that there was a lot of knowing hilarity about this advice and the permission it unwittingly gave to gay experiences. It was quite a large group with perhaps four people considering whether they were gay or bisexual; two of us now live with our same-sex partners.'

Alex encountered Christian attitudes to sex and relationships at a summer worship festival that he attended as a teenager. 'This festival was a huge part of my teenage faith,' he explains. 'I met with God in some profound ways there, memories of which kept my faith going through later, spiritually drier times at university. There was a clear focus on helping people to deal with all sorts of pastoral issues, but gay people were rarely mentioned. It was clear that relationships weren't an option for gay people, but how we were actually supposed to deal with that was never touched upon. Their position could be summed up as "God wants you to save yourself for marriage because he loves you and it's what is best for you".'

He finally drew his own conclusions, that, 'If the marker of appropriateness was what is "best for people", then there is no sensible reason why a committed, emotionally fulfilling gay relationship should be wrong.' This is similar to the belief that Michael came to, after plenty of thought and prayer: 'God doesn't want me to get hurt physically or emotionally, which is why he gave people rules and guidance. "Casual sex gets you hurt" is the underlying message of all the various sexual rules and regulations in the Bible.'

There are tools available to Christians for considering sexual ethics. By looking at the Bible and tradition afresh and reflecting together on our experience, we can start to explore our attitudes to same-sex relationships. This is an approach that Mark has taken. He's a straight man and self-proclaimed conservative evangelical, so you might not think him a natural advocate for same-sex relationships, but his reflection on the nature of relationship in the Bible has changed his mind on the acceptability of long-term same-sex relationships. His starting point is that, 'Fundamentally, Christianity is a religion whose basis is the loving relationship between God and humanity, and loving relationships between people. Examples of such long-term loving relationships include God's covenant with Israel, the commitment between fellow believers, parents and children, masters and servants, the commitment to foreigners, widows, orphans, and Jesus' commitment to us through the cross and through the Holy Spirit. Given the Bible's support for long-term relationships I gave up a theology whose implication would be to split couples (and therefore potentially parents and children) who had made long-term commitments to each other, for example through civil partnership/same-sex marriage.'

There are some formal statements of shared values about sexual relationships which refute the idea that 'anything goes', but are more complex than an unquestioning belief in 'no sex before marriage'. For example, a Methodist Conference resolution passed in 1993 maintains that 'all sexual practices, which are promiscuous, exploitative or demeaning, are unacceptable forms of behaviour and contradict God's purposes for us all'. This is only a starting point. John, who was present at the debate about this resolution, now believes that it's time for the church to give some positive guidance: 'It would be helpful if the church could describe wholesome relational behaviour such as love, respect, fairness, attentiveness, reciprocity and faithfulness which would be encouraged in any relationship – parent/child, between siblings, in both straight and gay relationships, before and after marriage/civil partnership. Sexual activity would be judged in so far as it is loving, respectful, fair, attentive and faithful.'

We can't resolve these big questions of sexual ethics here. You may read this section and think we should have taken a firmer line against sex outside permanent relationships. Others of you may think we should have done more to challenge straight cultural norms. Some of you will agree with our contributors, others will come to different conclusions. You yourself may be in a committed partnership, or happily or unhappily single. 'Lots of gay people are in perfectly happy, long-term, committed relationships,' Alex reminds us. 'And lots aren't. Just like straight people, in fact.'

Tying the knot

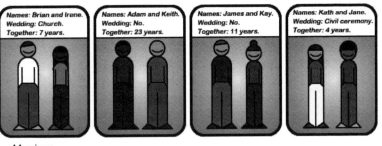

Marriage

You open your post one morning, and find an invite to a Civil Partnership Blessing/Same-Sex Wedding/Celebration of Civil Partnership. Civil partnerships are still fairly unusual, so you might be wondering what the day will be like and how to respond to that invite. Vivien (Rachel's mum), says that while she viewed Sarah as part of the family and thought that we 'would stay together in the long term', she had 'not really thought about marriage, or a wedding. At that time, the new civil partnership law was being discussed in Parliament, but I thought it would be a considerable time before this became law and just hoped that one day it would.' Now that it has, you'll be seeing plenty more same-sex couples tying the knot, so read on for the low-down on civil partnerships and same-sex weddings for friends, family, ministers, and of course for the happy couples themselves.

First, the boring legal stuff. In the UK until recently, mixed-sex couples could have a religious marriage service (in a church or other place of worship) which was also recognized legally. Alternatively, they could have a civil marriage (in a register office, hotel, football stadium, up the Blackpool Tower, etc.) which couldn't mention God at all. There was no legal recognition of their relationship for same-sex couples, although this did not stop them from having blessings or church services to recognize their relationship before God. However, because these weren't legal, they still had to write 'single' on tax returns and so on (told you this bit was boring!).

This all changed in 2005, when the Civil Partnership Act was passed, meaning that same-sex couples could now have the equivalent of a civil marriage, with a few inexplicable differences – for example the partnership becomes legally binding through the couple signing their names rather than by saying vows, and is called civil partnership rather than marriage. There's still no equivalent of religious marriage for same-sex couples, so while they can have a religious service, if they find a church willing to do it, for legal recognition they must have a civil partnership too.

In June 2008, the *Daily Telegraph* splashed news of what it called the 'Anglican Church's first gay "wedding"' across its front page. What the article described as 'shocking' and 'provocative' wasn't the relationship itself, but rather that two committed Christians had decided to celebrate their love in church, rather than simply with a civil partnership, and the implications that this could have for the wider church. The story and the reaction to it in the media sent a clear message to LGB people that they shouldn't expect a warm welcome from the church. The 'first gay wedding' also came as a surprise to those of us who had had our own hassle-free gay weddings many years before, but had forgotten to invite the press.

This media coverage showed that having a religious service alongside a civil partnership remains a step too far for some anti-LGB groups within the church. But times are constantly changing. Although these same people may have campaigned against the Civil Partnership Act, few now express outrage when same-sex couples celebrate a civil partnership as long as these couples do not expect their relationship to be blessed by the church. However, there are some couples for whom even having a secular civil partnership remains problematic. Sarah B, a lesbian priest, explains: 'My partner and I had already decided that we did not want to live together before we had made a formal commitment like civil partnership or marriage to each other. Heterosexual clergy couples are not allowed to live together prior to marriage, and we felt we should be held to the same standards. For the whole of our relationship, the UK has legally recognized same-sex relationships, but the bishop – and the majority of the church leadership – would not allow clergy to claim their civil rights and remain in parochial ministry.' As she explained in the previous chapter, Sarah B has found this pressure too much and soon she will be leaving parish ministry and moving with her partner to the USA. Only once she has left her job will they be able to mark their commitment to each other with a civil partnership in England and a religious ceremony in the States.

So, how important is the difference between civil and religious marriage? Well, for Christians, a wedding doesn't only mark the start of a contract or provide public recognition of a relationship. It is not about the perfect day, the perfect dress, the colour scheme and seeing how much you can spend. Many traditions describe it as a sacrament, the outward sign of an inward blessing, ordained by God, embedded in the history of the church and upheld by the Bible. They may even imply that marriage has been practised unchanging throughout the world and the centuries. Amen.

Same-sex couples have responded to these concepts of marriage in many different ways. Even though he believes the church should offer to bless same-sex relationships, Karl speaks for many, particularly older, LGB Christians when he explains why he would not want such a blessing himself: 'I do not believe we should attempt to copy "straight" society. Weddings are based on patriarchy and "romance". We should model alternative ways of relating.'

After all, marriage does not always get a good press. Some same-sex couples reject marriage because they perceive it to be oppressive to women, or simply irrelevant to their lives. They conclude that if the church doesn't welcome them as a same-sex couple, it makes little sense to go there to seek a blessing on or validation for their love. Some LGB people have already been in straight marriages before coming out, so marriage has difficult associations for them. Jo is one of them.

'For many years I stuck it out in a straight marriage because I thought I needed to deny myself,' she says. 'I thought I'd made my bed so needed to get on and lie in it. But I realized when I fell in love with a woman that my denial wasn't the Christian ideal I had hoped. I was instead denying myself and my husband a mutually fulfilling loving relationship. Living a lie was actually making me bitter and resentful and was taking me away from God. Now I'm being true to myself I can honestly strive to do what brings me closer to God.'

Marriage isn't the only rite of passage that our faith can offer couples; in any relationship, companionship and commitment are reflected in a hundred everyday ways, from sharing interests to sharing the housework. And they are reflected in significant milestones, like moving in together, taking responsibility for children or passing through a difficult and testing time side by side. Couples may want to mark these milestones, even if they do not want a marriage service. Sarah I and her partner had their house, garden and greenhouse blessed in a simple but meaningful ceremony that they devised with their vicar. This satisfied Sarah's desire for spiritual recognition of the relationship and was followed years later by a civil partnership. Sarah is adamant that any markers are stages along the journey and not an end in themselves. 'We recognize that our relationship is in a constant state of growth,' she says, 'and that our commitment has to be a process that is worked out day by day as we work at being lovers and love-bearers to one another and to all with whom we are connected.'

Bill had been with his partner for many years when he became ill with a suspected brain tumour. During his time in hospital, his partner would visit every day and they would attend Mass together in the hospital chapel. The chaplain offered Bill the sacrament of anointing for the sick for healing and wholeness (James 5.14). Unusually the chaplain also suggested anointing Bill's partner at the same time. 'There were some dozen people from our church in the hospital chapel, all there at very short notice, when we knelt side by side to be anointed,' he recalls. 'Our relationship was acknowledged and blessed sacramentally by the church acknowledging our vulnerability.'

This was not a marriage service in any traditional sense. Bill himself rejects that idea, saying that while their relationship is 'analogous to marriage in many ways, it is not marriage'. However, being offered a way to mark their relationship at such a traumatic time enabled them to publicly own and acknowledge its true depths, as strongly as any spoken vow to support each other 'in sickness and in health'. Later, Bill and his partner chose to register their civil partnership in a simple ceremony with just four witnesses, and 'unsentimental' vows that they wrote themselves, followed by a church blessing during the course of parish Mass.

If you are in a relationship with someone of a different faith or no faith at all, this may make focusing on a civil ceremony more appropriate. After her straight marriage ended and her relationship with her female partner blossomed, Jo was ready to embark on a civil partnership. 'We had a great day,' she explains. 'The only downside of the ceremony was not being able to use anything religious. Our spirituality is important to us. Even though we come from different faith traditions, at the level of spirituality and how we live it out, we have a lot more in common than people might think.' Despite this, they still found scope within their civil partnership ceremony to express their spirituality through poetry and readings. God can break out of the boundaries we set, and a civil partnership between two people who love each other can be infused with the presence and awareness of God, as can any church wedding, regardless of what words are said or sung.

Friends and family: how to respond to that invite

Our marriage was a pretty traditional occasion: a church service, an exchange of rings and of vows, prayers and hymns and a beaming bride in a big, white dress (hang on, was that two brides?). We started off by calling it a celebration, then a blessing and finally, as we and our minister grew more comfortable with the idea, simply our wedding.

If you are privileged enough to be invited to a friend or family member's same-sex wedding/blessing/celebration, then our advice is simple – relax. Whatever your views on the rights and wrongs of same-sex relationships, recognizing the significance of this commitment to someone you love is the best way to show them that you care about them.

If you feel unable to accept the invite, then quietly and calmly decline. Don't spend hours agonizing on the phone with the brides or grooms-to-be (as one of our friends did), as they have plenty of other things to worry about. Alternatively, think about whether there are parts of the event you feel able to support. We know of one couple with a Christian friend who felt that she couldn't in conscience attend their church service, but had no qualms with coming to the reception. Ideal – she helped to set up the venue and received deliveries while everyone else was in church.

Remember, it won't be as weird as you may imagine. The first same-sex wedding we went to was our own. We didn't know how it would feel to see, or to be, two women inhabiting a ceremony that has excluded LGB people in the past and is so associated with mixed-sex relationships. This is very likely to be how many guests feel too. After our wedding, a friend told us how strange she had thought the day would be, but on arrival soon forgot that it was any different from any other wedding. We recently received an invite from some friends which began, 'We realize that many of you will not have attended a same-sex blessing before, and that you may be slightly anxious or apprehensive about it. Please don't be,' before going on to explain clearly what to expect from the day. If you're not sure what you've been invited to and the information isn't on the invite, then find someone to ask.

Ministers: how to respond to a request to carry out the ceremony

In our experience, the biggest hurdle a same-sex couple is likely to encounter in planning their wedding is finding a church – and a minister – willing to host it. If you've been asked to do this, you may have given or considered one of these responses:

No.
I'd love to but . . .
   The bishop won't allow it.
   We're an ecumenical partnership and the others won't like it.
   The church isn't ready, maybe in a few years.
   I'm new to the church.
   I might lose my job.
   I've accepted the discipline of my church (even if I don't agree with it).
   We don't want the publicity.
   I'm washing my hair that day.

None of these are bad reasons, they come from trying to balance the needs of different people under your care and make difficult decisions about the best course of action. But they mean that people who want to form committed same-sex relationships may have to bear a disproportionate amount of the whole church's insecurity about relationships in a changing world. The cost for them is to see their relationships sidelined instead of celebrated and supported.

It is not easy to respond to the desire to give pastoral care; the knowledge that if you do you may face difficulties, and your own beliefs about what's right before God. Tony encountered this situation years ago and now looks back on his decision: 'Once, as a vicar, I was asked to bless the rings of a gay couple who had made a lifelong (but, at that time, unofficial) commitment to each other in love. I declined. I repent of that now. I cannot (yet?) affirm the absolute equality of gay and straight sexualities but I will, as a matter of Christian commitment, uphold the right of same-sex relationships to be accorded equal value and significance in the eyes of the church. If I was asked now, I would regard it as a privilege.'

Terry made a different decision when faced with a similar situation. 'When same-sex partnerships first became legal I was approached by a couple asking for a blessing. I agreed willingly, despite the fact that this would put my job on the line.' He explains the conviction that underpinned his decision: 'It's always angered me that I'm encouraged to bless war memorials, racehorses or motorway extensions, but am prevented from blessing two people in love who want to make a lifelong commitment before God.'

Tony and Terry will not be the only ministers to face such a dilemma. While a decreasing number of straight couples get married and two in every five of those marriages ends in divorce, same-sex couples are snapping up long-denied civil partnerships – over 18,000 in the first year alone. This has huge implications for the church and its clergy – what answers can we give to people who are looking for something more than a legal ceremony and who want to celebrate their love in a Christian context?

Even if you feel unable to hold a ceremony in your church, could you use the opportunity of being asked to do so to start conversations about same-sex relationships in your church? You might be able to reassure the couple that you'll 'turn a blind eye' to another minister carrying out the ceremony on your patch or find a way to support the couple that keeps your integrity – perhaps by leading a service in a garden, town hall function room or community centre, by agreeing a service that isn't like the traditional marriage service, or by saying some words at the start explaining this isn't a marriage according to the denominational rules. Or will you put your job on the line and lead an out-and-proud same-sex wedding, in your church, with bells ringing out the celebration across the parish, a full choir, vows, prayers and confetti? OK, skip the confetti if it's going to make a mess.

The happy couple: top tips to help plan your big day

You'll realize by now that if you want a church service to celebrate your same-sex partnership you should brace yourself for disappointment. We're sorry to say that unless you already know a minister who will help you, prepare for your request for a church blessing on your relationship to be refused. You will most likely be turned down kindly, but most ministers will turn you down. If you want an ordained minister, then be determined.

- **Start by asking your local parish priest or the leader of the church you attend** (their response might surprise you). But if that doesn't work, use insider knowledge: ask around your friends or contact any of the organizations listed on p. 161 and be prepared to try, try and try again. Rachel's mum showed admirable determination in finding a church for our wedding: 'I learnt not to take it personally, did not let the girls know how bigoted and intolerant I found some religious people, and soldiered on trying to find a church,' she says. 'I was determined that I would find one and refused to give up the search. If you really want something, don't give up.' And she succeeded!

- **Respect the risks.** If you do find a minister prepared to conduct the service and a church prepared to host it, appreciate that they may be taking a risk and could get into trouble with church authorities. Respect and discuss any need for privacy or sensitivities they have. We found our church and vicar separately, spreading and minimizing the risks to both. You may be unable to get married in the kind of church and in the kind of way you had always dreamed of. Think about how much this really matters, and where you are prepared to compromise.

- **Decide what you want the day to signify, and name it accordingly.** Some couples choose to use terms like 'friendship' or 'covenant relationship' rather than 'marriage' when marking their partnership publicly. These ideas are consistent with Christian tradition stretching back centuries, perhaps longer than romantic ideas of marriage common today, and are beautifully expressed in such biblical stories as David and Jonathan or Naomi and Ruth. They can be ideal for same-sex couples who want to avoid some of the baggage that comes with the concept of Christian marriage. We also like the way that Jo and her partner resolved the dilemma of what to call the occasion: 'We called our ceremony a civil partnership officially. To avoid heterosexual assumptions and stereotypes, we used the term wedding only with friends and family who would understand what we meant by it. But between the two of us, we thought of it as our big fat gay wedding!'

- **Seize the opportunity to do it your way.** Be as camp or as classy as you like. You can play it straight, by using the words and structure of the traditional marriage service – or you can introduce readings, prayers, music and symbols which are special to your journey as individuals and as a couple. You could write your own vows. The fact that there is no official liturgy and no legal form of words can free you up to devise a personally meaningful service. Books like

Geoffrey Duncan's *Courage to Love* (see 'Where to go next') are a rich source of material. It also means that if you hate the idea of being given away by your dad or having your best friend make an embarrassing speech, you don't have to do it! Planning the order of service in itself can bring out new depths in your relationship (or can end up in a slanging match over whether you'd rather walk down the aisle to 'Shine, Jesus, shine' or 'I am what I am').

- **Affirm and enjoy.** Realize the power of your example. Even though many more same-sex couples are publicly or semi-publicly celebrating their relationships in church, it is still unusual enough that if you do so, you will become a role model and an advertisement for 'gay marriage'. Your adult guests will be talking about your wedding at work the next day. Their children will be growing up in a world where same-sex relationships are visible, affirmed and perfectly normal. Very different from the world many of us grew up in. The daughter of one of Vivien's friends attended our wedding and had a fantastic time. Afterwards she told us it was the loveliest wedding she'd ever been to – although she later admitted that, at age 11, it was the first wedding of any kind she'd attended!

Whether you are thinking of embarking on a relationship, planning to tie the knot, or already celebrating many years of partnership, we wish you much happiness. The world has certainly changed. Paul T is one of the oldest contributors to this book and when he was growing up, homosexuality was illegal. But by the time civil partnerships had been introduced, he had been with his partner for over three decades and they were moving into retirement together. 'We did go through a civil ceremony when this became possible,' he says, 'not as a public act but rather for our own sake and with only a few friends. It is good to have done it.'

Spotlight on . . . arranging a gay wedding

'When Rachel told me that she and Sarah wanted to get married, would dearly love a church service and a reception in our garden, I was amazed. Once I got over the surprise I realized, to my joy, that I would be Mother of the Bride (albeit one of the brides), I could wear a big hat, and would be able to share in a very special ceremony for a very special daughter. It was now January and the girls wanted their wedding to take place in August followed by a civil partnership ceremony once it became law. There was a lot to be done.

'As I was aware that a church service was so important to the girls I took it upon myself to find a venue. My concern that they would not be discriminated against was also Rachel's concern for me when I contacted local churches. Rachel and Sarah had already found a minister who would conduct the service. So all I had to do was find the church! Not so easy. I talked to my village vicar who felt our village was not ready for this. In fact, when one of the churchwardens heard about the request he said 'over my dead body'.

'I learnt not to take such comments personally – *I was determined that I would find a church and refused to give up the search*. Then one vicar suggested I contact another, and that vicar suggested another and eventually I rang a Methodist minister, expecting to be given yet another person's name. But, no, joy of joys, he saw no problem at all and would discuss it at a church council meeting the next evening. And so we found the church. I was so grateful.

'The week before The Day we had a rehearsal and I was surprised how emotional I felt. The meaning of what was going to happen, the promise that my daughter was going to make to the person she loved, really impacted on me. I am sure that this is no different from any mother of the bride, but I also still had this nagging fear that something would happen, there would be a demonstration against gay weddings, against homosexuals – you name it, I feared it. But, unbeknown to me, two male gay friends of the girls had had the same thought and had offered to be bouncers, saying that they would deal with anything that went wrong. This was an enormous relief and I felt that I could relax a little.

'Why did I worry and spend nights wondering what would happen and not sleeping? Goodness knows, as in the end nothing did happen, not a single murmur. The church itself seemed to hold us and bestow love on the couple. Afterwards a close friend of mine said that she had never listened to the wedding vows and words in a service so much before, never been moved so much before, and never cried so much before at a wedding. I felt this summed it up for me; the event had been pioneering and felt so "right". My daughter had found the person she loved and wanted to spend the rest of her life with, wanted to demonstrate this love with friends in the sight of God, and had been able to do so. The heavens hadn't opened against her and us, and it felt as if God was giving the girls his blessing.'

Vivien

Action

Reflect on the weddings and civil partnerships that you've attended. Where did you find God in those occasions? How have they influenced your own relationship choices or hopes? Think about whether there are practical ways you can continue to support any of these couples and who you can find support from to help your own relationships to flourish.

Prayer

Loving God, thank you for those couples we know who have chosen the way of love and commitment. Strengthen, support and encourage them, we pray, so that what you have joined together, no one may put asunder. Amen.

9

Speaking out

Other people's awareness that my son was homosexual developed gradually because of conversations about family over coffee after morning service, items that I have written for parish or diocesan magazines, letters to newspapers, radio interviews and so on. An unexpected outcome has been that others within our congregation have shared with us that they too have family members, friends or colleagues who are gay. (Christine)

Whether it's bickering bishops, a papal pronouncement or an ill-advised comment from an evangelical leader, it's easy to find negative coverage of LGB issues and the church in the media. It may be true that conflict and controversy sell papers, but sadly these stories feed perceptions of Christianity as out of touch, sex-obsessed and hypocritical. The stories are themselves fed by other stereotypes, those of a 'gay lifestyle' of one-night stands and never managing to hold down any kind of stable relationship. They fall painfully short of addressing the complex reality of life as an LGB or LGB-affirming Christian.

Or there is simply silence. Fear of saying the wrong thing or of causing division means that LGB issues are seldom calmly and properly addressed within the church, and the spiritual needs and longings of LGB people and their families outside the church are largely ignored. We may find ourselves living a double life, hiding our faith from LGB friends who are hostile to Christianity or feeling that we constantly have to defend aspects of Christianity that we are not sure if we agree with ourselves.

Rather than giving up, it's up to us as LGB Christians, families, friends and allies to act positively and with passion. Our voices, actions and lives can tell a different story. This book is full of these kinds of stories.

Those around us are often more willing to listen than we realize. Now you've nearly reached the end of this book it's time to think about telling your stories and living your life to challenge and influence others. But how? As you'd expect by now, this final chapter is packed with contemporary wisdom from both LGB and straight Christians, but this time it's supplemented with biblical wisdom from the book of Proverbs.

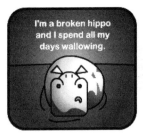 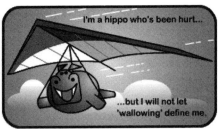

Commit to the LORD whatever you do and your plans will succeed (Proverbs 16.3)

As a priest and a lesbian, Sarah B regularly encounters uncertainty and hostility from people within the church about the ordination of women and of LGB people. As a result, she has had plenty of opportunities to speak out. She explains: 'I have been surprised by how many times someone has said to me, "We weren't sure about women priests, but you are OK", and then followed it by saying, "We couldn't have a gay priest."' While her gender is obvious to her parishioners, her sexual orientation is not. She faces a choice on each occasion about how to respond. 'My usual reply if I feel confident is "Maybe you've already experienced the ministry of a gay priest, and it's been OK too." Failing that, I say, 'Maybe in time your views will change."'

It can be hard to speak out against prevailing assumptions within a church. Accepting diversity and working to stop discrimination was part of the ethos of Ed's job in the police. He became a Christian in his forties and was full of the joys of his new-found faith when he started to witness individual and corporate discrimination against LGB friends in his church. 'I felt shocked that people who were proclaiming Jesus could be so seemingly unchristian. I found myself questioning my own faith and at one point was on the verge of cancelling my financial contributions to the church and looking for another one,' he says. 'Of course I didn't do these things. I took the coward's way out and told myself that I just needed to focus on Jesus and not get distracted by side issues. I have found myself not having the courage to be the dissenting voice when anti-gay opinions are raised in church circles. I must change this and learn to speak out when opportunities arise.'

Speaking out – or remaining silent – is not yet another thing to beat yourself up about. As Ed found, expressing a different view from the dominant one in a church can be especially difficult for new Christians. But it's still possible to be aware of opportunities that come along and use them in a loving way. Ed stood alongside and prayed with his LGB friends, letting others in the church see that he treated them just like everybody else. His actions showed his 'dissenting voice' even when he felt unable to speak out publicly.

There are many different ways to have an impact at a local level. Ruth and her partner approached their vicar to ask him to bless their new house. 'He's one of those vicars who's very nice,' she explains, 'but will spend a lot of time hand-wringing, worrying about the rest of the congregation. But he did come round to bless the house, and for him that is a step forward.' As a result of that encounter, one vicar has – perhaps for the first time – had to think about his engagement with LGB people and to take a small, but potentially risky, step in their support.

For those who feel confident enough to do so, Ruth suggests becoming a point of contact or role model in your church, so that 'if anyone comes through your church and needs help, they can be put in touch with you'. A simple offer, but one that could be a huge encouragement to others in that church.

When the righteous prosper, the city rejoices (Proverbs 11.10)

A few years ago when he was a student, Peter C joined a religious LGB group that had just been set up in his university. After several committee meetings and much thoughtful discussion, the group was given affiliated membership to an umbrella Christian organization: a small triumph in a city where the Christian Union held sway with a very traditional line.

However, Peter recalls, the press could not appreciate the progress that this showed, and seized on the fact that the group was given 'affiliated' rather than 'full' membership. 'It was a difficult journey for the umbrella Christian organization to accept an LGB group into membership in any way, and I think this was partly due to fear of press coverage,' he reflects now. 'Support of LGB people and organizations within the church is seen as antagonistic, rather than a pastoral success that should be celebrated publicly. For our part, LGB people can feel guilty for asking for any type of public endorsement, knowing that it may cause more division.'

During his forty years experience as a Methodist minister John has encountered this problem many times. He identifies it as the desire to keep the peace outweighing the thirst for justice. 'But if we can't have both the peace and the justice,' he wonders, 'are we willing to work for justice and risk the peace?'

His experience of working for justice and risking the peace has been mixed, but he has no regrets: 'When I have written in a local newspaper or church magazine or when I have raised issues of sexuality in worship or church meetings, I have received many appreciative comments from individuals. While some have taken issue with me, others have expressed great pleasure that "someone has been prepared to speak out".' Being that someone takes courage, and relies on the support of others. Those who have backed John and quietly expressed their support for his stance have a vital role in encouraging and affirming their more outspoken brothers and sisters.

Reckless words pierce like a sword, but the tongue of the wise brings healing (Proverbs 12.18)

Peter's experiences have taught him to recognize the roles that different people can play. He encourages straight Christians to speak out and LGB people to be ready to accept their support: 'When the debate flares up, the hopes of LGB people actually rest on straight Christians standing up for us, as our own opinions can always be dismissed as biased.' Elaine is one of these straight Christians who have signed petitions and written letters in support of LGB people within the church. But she suspects that 'the examples of godly life shown in many gay people, who are just getting on with things, will have a more persuasive effect than any flag-waving I might do'.

It is clearly effective to stand together. Like many straight people, Robyn finds that the struggle for an inclusive church is her struggle too: 'I feel genuinely ashamed of "the church is anti-gay" news stories. They undermine the Christian faith, both within and outside to non-Christians; misrepresent the church since many people (and I would say God!) are not anti-gay, and of course misrepresent gay people. There is a wider issue of a sensationalist and conflict-led media which perpetuates discrimination and sees people only as issues. It is this kind of attitude towards others that Christianity should stand against.'

Robyn believes that as the church becomes more welcoming and genuinely inclusive it becomes more Christian. This belief has inspired her to speak out: 'As a member of the Inclusive Church network and along with another straight friend, I wrote to all the churches in our Church of England diocese inviting them to sign up to the Inclusive Church statement of belief.' Putting your views down in writing as John and Robyn have done can be a positive way of building relationships, encouraging change and making sure that an anti-LGB perspective is not seen as the only one.

A few years ago a member of our then church, who also happens to be a high-profile evangelical leader, was quoted in the media opposing civil partnerships. We wrote a letter to him explaining how we found his comments difficult and suggesting we meet. A brief and awkward after-church chat followed. We didn't change our view and we're sure he didn't change his, but at least we had made personal contact. The other side of the debate now had a human face.

As Peter concludes: 'Now that media coverage has highlighted the LGB wound in the church, I suspect that we need less sensational, more personal communication to heal it.'

Pride breeds only quarrels, but wisdom is found in those who take advice (Proverbs 12.10)

If you are an Anglican, the chances are you will have heard something about the 'listening process', recommended by the Church's House of Bishops as a way forward in the debate about sexual orientation. Whether you feel this has been a catalyst for change or believe it has been largely ignored, genuinely listening to people's stories and experiences is vitally important. That's the case whatever tradition we come from, whether we oppose or support greater inclusion of LGB people or are simply confused.

But it's not easy. Alex explains that, in his experience, 'sometimes people are threatened by the fact that you don't think the same way as they do. Sometimes you might feel up for a fight, but if you're not, remember it's not your job to convince them. Many of us who are now gay-affirming took years to understand why the conservative position didn't make sense – those views are deeply ingrained in many Christians.'

After all, it is possible to listen to and understand someone else's views without having to abandon your own. This realization helped Sophie feel more comfortable with her LGB friends. She says, 'When my lesbian friend said that she wasn't necessarily expecting my views to change as a result of being friends with her, I think that helped me relax and just get on with being friends. It's possible to be friends with someone and not share their beliefs about everything.'

'I think that there are always going to be people who disagree, because that's what they genuinely believe,' adds Jim, who stopped attending church after being outed, but has since returned to worship. He continues: 'But in the church we can't be afraid to disagree with somebody. If you disagree accept that you disagree, don't make a big deal out of it. We've got to accept that people may think that what we do is wrong, but let them believe that for now, let's get them to accept us as people before anything else.' Even after genuinely listening to each other, it's only natural that differences of opinion will still exist, but relationships and attitudes towards individuals may start to shift. So many of the stories in this book bear witness to that truth.

Peter C puts listening in the context of love. 'Loving your neighbour as yourself', he believes, 'involves straight people listening fully to LGB people, and LGB people listening equally well to straight people. By talking about their sexuality to straight Christians, LGB Christians can help to dispel the myths that condemn us, and straight Christians, who have

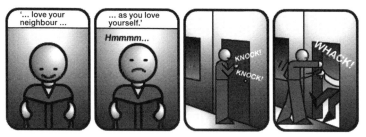

What can happen if you don't love yourself.

the much stronger position of being in the majority, can make sure there is support and space for LGB voices to be heard. Through this more thorough loving of our neighbours, we may be able to undo some of the hurt of the past and ensure that that wound is not continued into the future.'

A gentle answer turns away wrath, but a harsh word stirs up anger (Proverbs 15.1)

'I think the only time I really get interrogated about why I am a Christian is by gay people,' says Gwilym. 'Their assumptions about the way the church deals with gay people only characterize the most extreme experiences. I think that's a really sad thing, because that's the image the church as a whole has. It's important that we show that there are churches which are not like that and not every Christian feels that way.' But now other people have started asking him questions too: 'I was in the pub with a couple of people after work and my boss raised the subject. He said he only had what he saw in the media to go on, that seemed to say you can't be gay and Christian. But what really confused him was that I didn't do the two things separately; whenever I talked about a guy, somewhere in the story is the church, so he wanted to know where this "you can't be gay and Christian" thing came from. I had great difficulty answering that – there are so many issues to unpack I just didn't know where to start!'

Being LGB and a Christian does seem to open up opportunities for questions and discussions about faith that would not otherwise happen. Peter C has been 'surprised at the number of LGB people that I meet in secular settings who turn out to have a religious past and a strongly spiritual side. These people no longer attend their former religious establishments except for family occasions and their faith might seem to be dormant. However, I have hardly met any hostility when coming out as Christian, and my confession of faith often leads to an interesting conversation about what exactly people do believe, and also what aspects of the church they struggle with.' For him, these conversations even opened up the opportunity to write an article for a gay men's magazine about why Christianity was still relevant and important in today's world.

But sometimes, when those informal conversations lead to interaction with formal church structures, problems can start again. I (Rachel) ended up in an unexpected conversation about Christianity with a guest at a party. I explained to her that I had met the host through an LGB Christian group and as the night went on, the conversation deepened. As a result she signed up for an Alpha course at her local church. At the first session, after she had explained what had inspired her to come along, the leader told her that there was no such thing as an LGB Christian. She walked out of the course, and did not go back.

Speaking out doesn't necessarily mean sending out a press release, preaching a sermon or joining a campaign. It can mean simply listening to people who are cut off from or turned off by the institutional church, being open to questions and answering them honestly and patiently when they come.

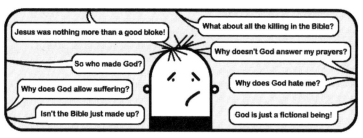

All I said was 'I'm a Christian.'

Even a child is known by their actions, whether their conduct is pure and right (Proverbs 20.11)

One of the clearest and most powerful ways of speaking out, Naomi explains, is to simply be yourself. She says: 'All I wanted was the choice of going out with who I wanted to. I didn't want this to be a big political statement, I just wanted to be who I was. But there are people I knew as a teenager who won't speak to me any more and there are other people who had their views challenged by what I was doing. Yet neither of those things was my intention. I didn't have to argue with other people to prove that I'm still a Christian. I still believe in God, and I haven't fundamentally changed. Just to live that out was really powerful.'

Telling stories, sharing personal experiences and living our lives with honesty and integrity are what this book is all about. Yet many contributors, like Paul B, have apologized about 'only' offering their story. 'I feel I am not really qualified, either personally as a heterosexual male, or theologically as someone who doesn't hold a theological degree,' he says. 'I can only relate my own story. I am sure the other contributors have better and more worthwhile stories to tell and points to make, but these experiences are valuable to me. They have helped teach me the value of vulnerability, of friendship, and also of how important it is to learn from each other with open minds and hearts. This, incidentally, strikes me as very biblical.'

While theological debate and campaigns to change church policy are vitally important, we believe that these values of vulnerability, friendship and openness are already transforming the church. Mark reminds us that, 'As Christians all of us are seeking to be salt and light to the people around us. My experience of church as a place for love, commitment and challenging of each other has been strengthened by engaging positively with gay Christians. Bridging the gay/straight fault line can be a great part of being a Christian, and I would encourage you to keep trying. We can all benefit from more friends.'

We are amazed by how willing the contributors to *Living It Out* have been to share their stories with us – and with you. Each story is unique, yet part of a bigger story in which we all share. We believe they can help 'bridge the gay/straight fault line' and give new insights into how LGB Christians, their families, friends and churches can not just survive, but flourish. We hope that *Living It Out* has helped you to understand your own story better and to continue living out your faith with boldness and with joy.

Action

Each previous chapter has ended with an action. If you're anything like us, you'll add this book to your shelf of Christian books without having done any of the actions. Why not go back now, choose one and actually do it?

Prayer

At home and at church, in reflection and in action, in our brokenness and in our striving for restoration, with love and with peace, may we go out and serve the Lord. Amen.

Where to go next: list of resources

The resources listed below, including websites, organizations and books, have all been recommended by our contributors. We hope you too will find these helpful, although we cannot personally vouch for those which we haven't visited, experienced or read. This list is by no means exhaustive, but gives a flavour of what's out there and how to get it. All details are correct at time of writing but if some change, an internet search engine should help you find up-to-date information.

Websites

www.livingitout.com

You've read the book, now visit the website. Here you can add your comments on *Living It Out*, find out more about the book and access further sources of support or information.

http://gaychristian.net

'An international, but USA-based community. The website has some helpful resources discussing the morality of same-sex relationships from an affirming evangelical perspective, has an active discussion forum, and some good podcasts.'
Recommended by Peter H.

www.religioustolerance.org

Nielsen's Links to Psychology and Religion Sites describes this site as giving 'information about many different religions, religion in the media and controversial topics. Probably the best site of its kind, and well worth your visit.' We agree.

www.smallpilgrimplaces.org.uk

'For breathing spaces on the pilgrim journey.'
Recommended by Gwilym.

Organizations

In general, we've listed organizations' websites and email contacts here, but most will have postal and phone contacts as well.

Affirmation Scotland

www.affirmationscotland.org.uk/index.html,
info@affirmationscotland.org.uk
Seeks the affirmation and dignity of LGB Christians in the Church of Scotland, provides worship and fellowship.

AXIOS: Eastern and Orthodox Gay and Lesbian Christians

www.eskimo.com/~nickz/axios.html
Recommended by Bill.

Centre for the Study of Christianity and Sexuality

www.cscs.co.uk
Publications and conferences.
Recommended by Paul T.

Changing Attitude England

www.changingattitude.org.uk, office@changingattitude.org
Network of lesbian, gay, bisexual, transgender and hetero-sexual members of the Church of England whose concern is to work for change in the church's understanding of human sexuality. Diocesan groups and events.
Recommended by Margaret.

Courage

www.courage.org.uk, office@courage.org.uk
Meetings and resources for gay and lesbian Christians seeking a safe place of friendship in which to reconcile their faith and sexuality and grow towards Christian maturity. Partners, friends, parents and other family members also welcome.
Led by one of our contributors Jeremy Marks.

The Evangelical Fellowship of Lesbian and Gay Christians (EFLGC)

www.eflgc.org.uk, info@eflgc.org.uk
Regular meetings, newsletter.

Families and Friends of Lesbians and Gays (FFLAG)

National Helpline 0845 6520311, www.fflag.org.uk,
info@fflag.org.uk
Support groups across the UK.
Recommended by Christine.

Inclusive Church

www.inclusivechurch2.net
An organization 'committed to ensuring that those who are excluded from the Anglican Communion because of their poverty, different abilities, ethnic origin or any other reason can play their full part in the gospel of Jesus Christ's unconditional love'.

Iona Community

www.iona.org.uk, ionacomm@iona.org.uk
'The liturgy, songs and writings of the people associated with the Iona Community are extremely helpful.'
Recommended by Jo.

Lesbian and Gay Christian Movement (LGCM)

www.lgcm.org.uk, lgcm@lgcm.org.uk
National membership organization with local groups.
Recommended by Paul T.

Metropolitan Community Church (MCC)

www.mccchurch.org, info@mccchurch.net
Christian denomination 'at the vanguard of civil and human rights movements and addresses the important issues of racism, sexism, homophobia, ageism and other forms of oppression'. It has 300 local congregations around the world, including in the UK.
Recommended by Kate.

Modern Churchpeople's Union

www.modchurchunion.org, office@modchurchunion.org
Anglican membership association which promotes liberal theology.
Recommended by Margaret.

Outcome

www.outcomeonline.org.uk
A group of LGBT ordained and lay Christians and their supporters in the Methodist Church.

OuterSpace at the Greenbelt Festival

www.greenbelt.org.uk, info@greenbelt.org.uk
www.outerspacelgbt.org.uk
Greenbelt is a Christian arts festival which takes place every August bank holiday at Cheltenham Racecourse. OuterSpace puts on LGBT-themed events at the Greenbelt Festival each year.

The Quakers

www.quaker.org.uk, outreach@quaker.org.uk
'Having been at a Quaker meeting for several years, I think that any LGB person will find it quite a comfortable environment. It gives everybody space to be their own person which I found extremely refreshing. LGB people are welcome like everybody else to assume positions of leadership.'
Recommended by David.

Quest

www.questgaycatholic.org.uk Helpline: 0808 808 0234
Group for lesbian and gay Catholics, local groups, bulletin and annual conference.
Recommended by Paul T.

YLGC – Young Lesbian, Gay, Bisexual and Transgender Christians

www.ylgc.org.uk, ylgc_group@yahoo.co.uk
UK-wide group for LGBT Christians aged 16 to 30. Regular meetings, online forum.
Recommended by several contributors.

Lists of LGB-friendly churches

These local churches that have made a public commitment saying that they welcome LGB people are sometimes called inclusive churches or affirming congregations. As far as we are aware, lists are only available for the Anglican Church and the Church of Scotland at the moment. You can also use the links below to find out how to add your church to the list.

Anglican Church

www.inclusivechurch2.net/Churches-Books-Resources-f7b16ae
www.changingattitude.org.uk/welcong/welcongs.asp

Church of Scotland

www.affirmationscotland.org.uk/congregations.htm

Books

Faith Beyond Resentment: Fragments Catholic and gay
by James Alison (Darton, Longman and Todd)

'This book took me on a journey on which I met with my own brokenness and tears at my sense of being understood. Reading this was not an experience merely of recognizing some of the sentiments expressed, or of enjoying an engaging read. It was like reading my own thoughts, my own situation, my own excruciating pain, written more clearly than I could ever have thought; let alone expressed.'
Recommended by Richard P.

On Being Liked by James Alison (Darton, Longman and Todd)

'This book refers once again to the church's double-binds that leave gay people living death: Love/Do not love. Be (all that you were made to be)/Do not be. Alison argues that as the church wrestles with matters of sexuality, the authentically catholic question is not 'What would Jesus do?' but instead 'What is Jesus doing?' While we (with many perspectives) in the church find ourselves scandalized, we have missed that the gospel is supposed to be about the undoing of scandal. James Alison is no easy read, intellectually or emotionally, but is worth the journey.'

Recommended by Richard P.

The Marriage of Likeness: Same-sex unions in pre-modern Europe by John Boswell (Fontana Press)

Recommended by Terry.

Sodomy: A history of a Christian biblical myth by Michael J. Carden (Equinox Publishing)

'A superb analysis of the true meaning of the stories of Sodom and Gomorrah.'
Recommended by Terry.

Gay Theology Without Apology by Gary David Comstock (Pilgrim Press)

Recommended by Aidan.

Good Fruits: Same-sex relationships and Christian faith
Pleasure, Pain and Passion: Some perspectives on
sexuality and spirituality
both by Jim Cotter (Cairns Publications)

Recommended by Terry.

The Other Way? Anglican lesbian and gay journeys
edited by Colin Coward (Changing Attitude)

Recommended by Terry.

Courage to Love: An anthology of inclusive worship material compiled by Geoffrey Duncan (Darton, Longman and Todd)

'A timely and moving anthology which will provide strength and inspiration to those who want to celebrate their God-given sexuality in the face of continuing rejection and hostility.' *Recommended by Christine.*

Reluctant Journey: A pilgrimage of faith from homophobia to Christian love by George Hopper (can be downloaded from www.reluctantjourney.co.uk)

Recommended by Christine.

A Churchless Faith by Alan Jamieson (SPCK Publishing)

'Research about why people leave Evangelical, Pentecostal and Charismatic churches in New Zealand. I found it to be a very helpful account of spiritual development or stages of faith and how growth often involves a time away from church.' *Recommended by Sophie.*

The Meaning in the Miracles by Jeffrey John (Canterbury Press)

'My all-time favourite biblical commentary, it is also so much more. It unpacks the great riches in the miracle stories of the Gospels in a way that is tremendously well informed, yet fresh and vital. One of the chapters does deal specifically with "the gay issue" in the story of the healing of the centurion's servant. But, far more important it seems to me is the spirit of life-affirming inclusion that permeates the book and the wide variety of quotations for reflection at the end of each chapter. I turn to it for help for many different reasons and it is a great reminder why we think this man Jesus is worth following in the first place.' *Recommended by Elaine.*

Permanent, Faithful, Stable by Jeffrey John (Darton, Longman and Todd)

'This hardly needs my commendation as best of the books for a thoughtful, readable look at Christian same-sex partnerships, covering many "old chestnut" issues. The three sections (Is it scriptural? Is it moral? Is it achievable?) reveal the structure and weight of this little book.'
Recommended by Richard P.

The Revelations of Divine Love by Julian of Norwich (Penguin Classics)

'The quality that books like this have is that they dwell on the positive, whereas so much religion does exactly the opposite. By surrounding you with such a positive sense of the love of God, they invoke a response from you that brings out the best in you and enables you (among other things) to deal with the negative within yourself naturally, constructively and without undue emphasis. Julian makes you feel that you are worth something, that God really values you, rather than standing over you with an angry temper and a whip; she makes you feel that God's love is actually reaching you, rather than just being something remote which you are sick of hearing the local parish jobsworth going on about.'
Recommended by David.

No Ordinary Child: A Christian mother's acceptance of her gay son by Jacqueline Ley (Wildgoose Publications)

Recommended by Terry.

Good Goats: Healing our image of God by Dennis, Sheila and Matthew Linn (Paulist Press International)

'This book describes a theology of God as loving and not vengeful. A helpful book for getting over harsh visions of God,

and realizing that there are orthodox views which are more loving and forgiving than the conservative evangelical view.'
Recommended by Sophie.

A New Kind of Christian by Brian D MacLaren (Jossey Bass)

'Where I began to find alternative structures for my thoughts about faith.'
Recommended by Richard P.

Towards a Theology of Gay Liberation edited by Malcolm Macourt (SCM Press)

Recommended by Terry.

The Bell by Iris Murdoch (Penguin Books)

'This novel gives a reflective approach to the question of same-sex desire and Christian discipleship. Although some of its assumptions now seem out of date, it nevertheless offers insights into the internal struggles that many LGB Christians continue to face. As such, it rings true (no pun intended), allows one to observe these psychological and spiritual phenomena from the outside, and helps one to feel less alone.'
Recommended by Daniel.

In the Eye of the Storm by Gene Robinson (Canterbury Press)

'Here, Gene Robinson tells his story. He reflects on his journey of faith, the scandal his election has caused to some and the affirmation and hope it has brought to countless others who, in various ways, find themselves on the margins of today's world.'
Recommended by Christine.

Sexuality and the Christian Body: Their way into the Triune God by Eugene F. Rogers (Blackwell)

'Interacting imaginatively with the theology of Thomas Aquinas and Karl Barth, Rogers argues that God's dealings with the church are "unnatural" – a word all too commonly reserved for same-sex desire alone, à la St Paul in Romans 1. Far from standing in the way of grace, however, bodies and sexuality are a means to it. And nowhere is this more evident than in a community (be it monastic or matrimonial) whose members provide an environment in which each can flourish.'
Recommended by Daniel.

Everything belongs: The gift of contemplative prayer by Richard Rohr (Crossroad Publishing Company)

Recommended by Jo.

Daring to Speak Love's Name: A gay and lesbian prayer book by Elizabeth Stuart (Hamish Hamilton)

Recommended by Terry.

Gay and Lesbian Theologies: Repetitions with critical difference by Elizabeth Stuart (Ashgate)

Recommended by Bill.

Just Good Friends: Towards a theology of lesbian and gay relationships by Elizabeth Stuart (Continuum)

Recommended by Aidan.

The Savage Text: The use and abuse of the Bible by Adrian Thatcher (Wiley-Blackwell)

'This book asks how Christians have been able to conduct, in public and on a global scale, arguments which have exposed

so much hatred and misrepresentation that the very mission of the church has been severely compromised.'
Recommended by Christine.

The Post-Evangelical by Dave Tomlinson (Triangle)

'Although a few years old now, begins to deconstruct some of the evangelical baggage that many of us have grown up with.'
Recommended by Richard P.

Strangers and Friends: New exploration of homosexuality and the Bible by Michael Vasey (Hodder and Stoughton)

Recommended by Bill.

Inspiration from the Bible . . .

'As encouragement for those who suffer ill-treatment from church officials (for any reason) I love the **History of Susanna; (from the Apocrypha, or Daniel 13 in the Catholic version of the Bible).** Susanna is a lovely spiritual woman who wants to be her best for God, and who is taken advantage of by a couple of religious elders who, for their own purely selfish motives, try to stitch her up. Then along comes Daniel, exposes publicly what they are doing, the elders get their just deserts and Susanna emerges with quiet and triumphant dignity.'
Recommended by David.

. . . And a final word on choosing books

'If you feel like you are wrestling through life, read anything else that will relieve the weight on your shoulders. Just find any way you can to laugh. Many of us Christians have come to take ourselves rather too seriously, which is a significant part of the church's problems. A Christian housemate once told me that she didn't read anything but Christian books. I was horrified. And soon after I came out.'
Recommended by Richard P.

General Index

Index of Biblical References